Vascular Surgical Emergencies

Susanne Regus

Vascular Surgical Emergencies

Well-Prepared for Duty

Springer

Susanne Regus
Bamberg, Germany

ISBN 978-3-662-72645-7 ISBN 978-3-662-72646-4 (eBook)
https://doi.org/10.1007/978-3-662-72646-4

Translation from the German language edition: "Gefäßchirurgische Notfälle" by Susanne Regus, © Der/die Herausgeber bzw. der/die Autor(en), exklusiv lizenziert an Springer-Verlag GmbH, DE, ein Teil von Springer Nature 2025. Published by Springer Berlin Heidelberg. All Rights Reserved.

This book is a translation of the original German edition "Gefäßchirurgische Notfälle" by Susanne Regus, published by Springer-Verlag GmbH, DE in 2025. The translation was done with the help of an artificial intelligence machine translation tool. A subsequent human revision was done primarily in terms of content, so that the book will read stylistically differently from a conventional translation. Springer Nature works continuously to further the development of tools for the production of books and on the related technologies to support the authors.

This Springer imprint is published by the registered company Springer-Verlag GmbH, DE, part of Springer Nature.
The registered company address is: Heidelberger Platz 3, 14197 Berlin, Germany

Contents

Part I
My First Shift in Vascular Surgery

1 Emergency Situations in Vascular Surgery—The Top 22

The following lists 22 emergency situations, each with possible diagnoses. Details on the diagnoses can be found in the respective chapters.

Emergency Situation	Details in the following chapters
Aneurysms	• Ruptured popliteal aneurysm • Carotid artery rupture • Acute carotid dissection • Ruptured abdominal aortic aneurysm (rAAA) • Ruptured iliac aneurysm (rIA) • Acute aortic dissection • Leriche syndrome • Septic aortic erosion bleeding • Ruptured visceral artery aneurysm
Abdominal pain	• Ruptured abdominal aortic aneurysm (rAAA) • Ruptured iliac aneurysm (rIA) • Acute aortic dissection • Leriche syndrome • Septic aortic erosion bleeding • Mesenteric infarction • Ruptured visceral artery aneurysm • Portal vein thrombosis • Mesenteric vein thrombosis • Ischemic colitis after aortic procedures

S. Regus, *Vascular Surgical Emergencies*,
https://doi.org/10.1007/978-3-662-72646-4_1

Emergency Situation	Details in the following chapters
Bleeding	• Septic erosion bleeding • Pseudoaneurysm of the carotid artery • Pseudoaneurysm in the groin after puncture • Anastomotic aneurysm in the groin • Ruptured popliteal aneurysm • Shunt bleeding • Traumatic aortic rupture • Carotid artery rupture • Vascular trauma with foreign body in situ • Avulsion of the axillary artery • Avulsion of the brachial artery • Avulsion of the popliteal artery • Ruptured abdominal aortic aneurysm (rAAA) • Ruptured iliac aneurysm (rIA) • Septic aortic erosion bleeding • Ruptured visceral artery aneurysm • Rebleeding
Dialysis patients	• Peripheral arterial occlusive disease (PAOD) stage IV • Jugular vein thrombosis • Phlegmon of the lower leg • Sepsis due to toe gangrene • Infection of atrial catheter • Phlegmon of the lower leg • Shunt occlusion • Shunt bleeding • Shunt infection
Vascular trauma	• Pseudoaneurysm of the carotid artery • Pseudoaneurysm in the groin after puncture • Shunt bleeding • Traumatic aortic rupture • Carotid artery rupture • Vascular trauma with foreign body in situ • Avulsion of the axillary artery • Avulsion of the brachial artery • Avulsion of the popliteal artery • Acute carotid dissection • Acute aortic dissection • Rebleeding • Compartment syndrome

Emergency Situation	Details in the following chapters
Infections	• Septic erosion bleeding • Pseudoaneurysm in the groin after puncture • Anastomotic aneurysm in the groin • Peripheral arterial occlusive disease (PAOD) stage IV • Thrombophlebitis of the arm veins • Phlegmon of the lower leg • Foot abscess in diabetics • Acute Charcot foot • Sepsis due to toe gangrene • Port catheter infection • Infection of atrial catheter • Shunt bleeding • Shunt infection • Phlegmon of the lower leg • Septic aortic erosion bleeding • Ruptured visceral artery aneurysm • Bypass infection
Ischemia	• Ruptured popliteal aneurysm • Acute arterial occlusion of the leg • Acute arterial occlusion of the arm • Phlegmasia coerulea dolens • Avulsion of the axillary artery • Avulsion of the brachial artery • Avulsion of the popliteal artery • Symptomatic carotid stenosis • Acute carotid occlusion • Acute carotid dissection • Acute aortic dissection • Leriche syndrome • Mesenteric infarction • Portal vein thrombosis • Bypass occlusion • Bypass infection • Ischemic colitis after aortic procedures • Rebleeding • Compartment syndrome
Emergencies in anesthesia	• Septic erosion bleeding • Pseudoaneurysm of the carotid artery • Pseudoaneurysm in the groin after puncture
Emergencies in cardiology	• Pseudoaneurysm in the groin after puncture • Acute arterial occlusion of the leg • Acute arterial occlusion of the arm • Phlegmon of the lower leg • Acute aortic dissection

Emergency Situation	Details in the following chapters
Emergencies in nephrology	• Pseudoaneurysm in the groin after puncture • Peripheral arterial occlusive disease (PAOD) stage IV • Jugular vein thrombosis • Phlegmon of the lower leg • Infection of atrial catheter • Shunt occlusion • Shunt bleeding • Shunt infection
Emergencies in neurology/ neuro-radiology	• Pseudoaneurysm of the carotid artery • Pseudoaneurysm in the groin after puncture • Symptomatic carotid stenosis • Acute carotid occlusion • Acute carotid dissection • Postoperative carotid occlusion
Emergencies in Trauma Surgery	• Traumatic aortic rupture • Carotid artery rupture • Vascular trauma with foreign body in situ • Axillary artery avulsion • Brachial artery avulsion • Popliteal artery avulsion • Acute carotid dissection • Compartment syndrome
Emergencies in Urology	• Ruptured abdominal aortic aneurysm (rAAA) • Ruptured iliac aneurysm (rIA)
Emergencies in Visceral Surgery	• Mesenteric infarction • Ruptured visceral artery aneurysm • Portal vein thrombosis • Mesenteric vein thrombosis • Ischemic colitis after aortic procedures • Burst abdomen • Compartment syndrome
Postoperative Complications	• Septic erosion bleeding • Pseudoaneurysm in the groin after puncture • Anastomotic aneurysm in the groin • Port catheter dysfunction • Port catheter infection • Atrial catheter infection • Shunt occlusion • Shunt bleeding • Shunt infection • Septic aortic erosion bleeding (stent/bypass) • Postoperative carotid occlusion • Bypass occlusion • Phlegmon of the lower leg • Bypass infection • Rebleeding • Ischemic colitis after aortic procedures • Burst abdomen • Compartment syndrome

Emergency Situation	Details in the following chapters
Strokes	• Carotid artery pseudoaneurysm • Traumatic aortic rupture • Carotid artery rupture • Axillary artery avulsion • Symptomatic carotid stenosis • Acute carotid occlusion • Acute carotid dissection • Acute aortic dissection • Postoperative carotid occlusion
Shunts	• Thrombophlebitis of arm veins • Atrial catheter infection • Shunt occlusion • Shunt bleeding • Shunt infection
Veins and Venous Access	• Thrombophlebitis of arm veins • Deep vein thrombosis of the leg • Axillary/arm vein thrombosis • Jugular vein thrombosis • Phlegmasia coerulea dolens • (Ascending) thrombophlebitis of the saphenous vein • Thrombophlebitis of the small saphenous vein • Port catheter dysfunction • Port catheter infection • Shunt occlusion • Portal vein thrombosis • Mesenteric vein thrombosis • Compartment syndrome
Vital Emergencies	• Septic erosion bleeding • Pseudoaneurysm in the groin after puncture • Thrombophlebitis of arm veins • Phlegmasia coerulea dolens • Shunt bleeding • Traumatic aortic rupture • Carotid artery rupture • Vascular trauma with foreign body in situ • Popliteal artery avulsion • Acute carotid occlusion • Ruptured abdominal aortic aneurysm (rAAA) • Ruptured iliac aneurysm (rIA) • Acute aortic dissection • Leriche syndrome • Septic aortic erosion bleeding • Mesenteric infarction • Ruptured visceral artery aneurysm • Rebleeding • Compartment syndrome

Emergency Situation	Details in the following chapters
Soft Tissue Infections	• Phlegmon of the lower leg • Foot abscess in diabetics • Phlegmon of the lower leg • Acute Charcot foot • Sepsis due to toe gangrene
Toe Gangrene	• Peripheral arterial occlusive disease (PAOD) stage IV • Foot abscess in diabetics • Acute Charcot foot • Sepsis due to toe gangrene • Leriche syndrome • Phlegmon of the lower leg
Central Venous Catheters	• Axillary/arm vein thrombosis • Jugular vein thrombosis • Port catheter dysfunction • Port catheter infection • Atrial catheter infection • Shunt infection

2 Well Prepared for Duty

2.1 Medications

Below is a list of what I consider to be the most important medications and their dosages. This list is generally sufficient in > 80% of cases to manage a shift. Special and institution-specific medications should be added as needed. Space has been provided for your own notes and additions for this purpose.

Pain Medication

- **Metamizole (Novalgin®)**
  - 4 × 20–40 drops (gtt) or
  - 4 × 500–1000 mg i.v./p.o.
- **Paracetamol (Benuron®, Paracetamol ratio®)**
  - 4 × 500–1000 mg i.v./p.o.
- **Piritramide (Dipidolor®)**
  - 1–2 ampoules (15 mg each) s.c./i.v. up to 4 × daily
- **Tilidine/Naloxone (Valoron®×; Tilidin comp®)**
  - 50 mg/4 mg (Valoron®) up to 8 × daily
  - 100 mg/8 mg (Tilidin comp®) up to 4 × 1 tablet or
  - 20 (= 50 mg) to 40 (=100 mg) drops up to 4 (–8) × daily
- **Oxycodone/Naloxone (Oxycocomp®)**
  - 20 mg/10 mg up to 4 × 1 tablet
- **Morphine (Capros®)**
  - 10–20 mg p.o. 1–0–1 (up to 60 mg)
  - 5–10 mg i.m./s.c. 1–1–1–1
  - 1–2 mg/h via perfusor (1 mg/ ml, infusion rate 1–2 ml/h)

S. Regus, *Vascular Surgical Emergencies*,
https://doi.org/10.1007/978-3-662-72646-4_2

Antibiotics

- **Piperacillin/Tazobactam (e.g., Tazobac®)**
  - 4 g/0.5 g 1–1–1(–1)
- **Meropenem (e.g., Meronem®)**
  - 1 g 1–1–1(–1)
  - Clindamycin (e.g., Sobelin®, Clinda®)
  - 600 mg 1–1–1(–1)

Coagulation Optimization

- **Phytomenadione (Konakion®)**
  - for coagulation disorder under phenprocoumon
  - 2–5 mg
    Ampoules usually contain 1 mg/0.1 ml
    2 mg ampoules (0.2 ml) and 10 mg ampoules (1 ml)
    1 drop = 0.05 ml
    2 drops = 0.1 ml = 1 mg
- **PCC (Beriplex®)**
  - for emergency indication
  - Prothrombin (Factor II), Proconvertin (Factor VII), Stuart-Prower factor (Factor X), antihemophilic factor B (Factor IX)
  - Formula for required units:
    Target Quick (%) minus lab Quick (%) × body weight (kg)
  - Maximum dose 5000 IU
- **Protamine hydrochloride (Protamin ME®)**
  - for rebleeding and/or heparin overdose
  - 5000 IU/ml
  - 1 IU antagonizes 1 IU heparin

Anticoagulation

- **Unfractionated heparin**
  - 500–1000 IU/h via perfusor
  - Dosage scheme for a perfusor syringe (50 ml)
    5 ml heparin = 25000 IU with
    45 ml NaCl
      yields 500 IU/ ml
    Infusion rate
      1 ml/h = 500 IU
      2 ml/h = 1000 IU
  - PTT (partial thromboplastin time) monitoring every 6–12 h, target value 60–80 sec.

Practical Tip

- If coagulation parameters are within the normal range, start with 1000 IU/h
- Check after 6 hours, then every 12 hours
- If PTT = target range, maintain infusion rate

- If PTT < target range, increase infusion rate by 0.5 ml/h
- If PTT > target range, decrease infusion rate by 0.5 ml/h

- **Low-molecular-weight heparin**
  - weight-adjusted
  - e.g., enoxaparin (Clexane®) 1 mg/kg body weight 2 × daily
    Prefilled syringes 1 mg = 0.01 ml = 100 IU
    e.g., Clexane® 40 ≙ 40 mg ≙ 0.4 ml ≙ 4000 IU
    Clexane® 20/40/60/80/100 (each in mg) available
- **Fondaparinux (Arixtra®)**
  - Heparinoid
  - synthetically produced, parenterally administered pentasaccharide
  - prophylactic dose 2.5 mg 1 × daily s.c.
  - therapeutic dose 7.5 mg 1 × daily s.c.
- **Rivaroxaban (Xarelto®)**
  - Day 1–20: 15 mg 2 × daily
  - from day 21: 20 mg 1 × daily
- **Dabigatran (Pradaxa®)**
  - 150 mg 2 × daily (2 × 110 mg > 80 years and CrCl <30)
- **Apixaban (Eliquis®)**
  - Day 1–7: 10 mg 2 × daily
  - from day 8: 5 mg 2 × daily
- **Edoxaban (Lixiana®)**
  - 60 mg 1 × daily
- **Phenprocoumon (Marcumar®)**
  - according to coagulation values

Practical tip
- Start with 3–2–1, then check coagulation
- Quick 20–30%/INR 2–3
- Overlapping heparin administration is necessary until the target range is reached, because:
  - thrombophilia at the start of anticoagulation and
  - risk of "Marcumar necrosis"

Rheologics
- **Alprostadil = Prostaglandin E (Prostaglandin®)**
  - 2 × 40 μgt as short infusion

Platelet aggregation inhibition
- **Acetylsalicylic acid 100 mg (ASA®)**
  - 100 mg 1 × daily
- **Clopidogrel 75 mg (Plavix®)**
  - 75 mg 1 × daily (if ASA® intolerance)

- **Prasugrel (Efient®)**
  - 10 mg 1 × daily
  - Loading dose 60 mg
  - 5 mg 1 × daily, if
    > 75 years or
    < 60 kg

Renal insufficiency

- **CPS® powder (poly(styrene-co-divinylbenzene)sulfonic acid, calcium salt)**
  - for hyperkalemia
  - 1 sachet (= 15 mg) 1–4 × daily

Thrombolytics

- **rtPA ("recombinant tissue plasminogen activator") (Actilyse®)**
  - for arterial occlusions
  - for shunt occlusion
  - Ampoules: 2/10/20/50 mg
  - mix with heparin
  - Single dose 5 (–10 mg)
    1 mg + 1000 IU heparin
    5 mg + 5000 IU heparin

2.2 Lab Coat Pocket

Making phone calls is part of the daily and nightly routine on duty. There is hardly anything more unpleasant (on duty) than being in the middle of an emergency treatment and not having the phone numbers of important contacts at hand or having to search for them first. Not being able to make outgoing calls because the code for external call authorization is unknown is also a classic scenario during your first shifts. Therefore, after some nerve-wracking experiences, I have made it a habit to find out these numbers in advance to be prepared for critical situations.

Here is a list of important aids and work tools for your lab coat pocket, with space for your own notes and additions.

Tools and work equipment	
	List with all important telephone numbers
	This book, possibly as an eBook
	Current duty roster
	Cell phone (to Durern's chagrin...)
	Doppler
	Possibly portable s sono device (if available)

Part II
Arterial Bleeding

Septic Erosive Bleeding

3

Septic erosion bleeding preferentially affects vascular anastomoses following alloplastic reconstructions. It most commonly occurs in the groin area, but a "bio-patch" can also become infected and, if in doubt, must be explanted and replaced autologously (using a vein).

Case Example
67-year-old patient with known alcohol and nicotine abuse, history of femoral endarterectomy and patch plasty (synthetic material) 6 months ago, known secondary wound healing, wounds finally healed for 4 weeks. Now presents to the emergency department with massive, sudden swelling and redness in the groin, fever and chills for 3 days, CTA shows a large aneurysm in the operated groin with active bleeding into the tissue (Fig. 3.1), skin still intact but severe tenderness and already visible tension blisters. What would you do?

Definition
- Infection-induced erosion of a vessel, usually at the site of anastomoses
- Often chronic with the formation of a fistula or also
- acute bleeding complication

Typical Patient
- Usually a known patient with a recent or historical peripheral or central alloplastic bypass
- Often also with a previous patch plasty
- frequently groin, as this is where the highest germ density is found!
- sometimes previous puncture of a postoperative seroma (which should be strongly discouraged)
- usually synthetic replacement, but also possible with xenogeneic material

S. Regus, *Vascular Surgical Emergencies*,
https://doi.org/10.1007/978-3-662-72646-4_3

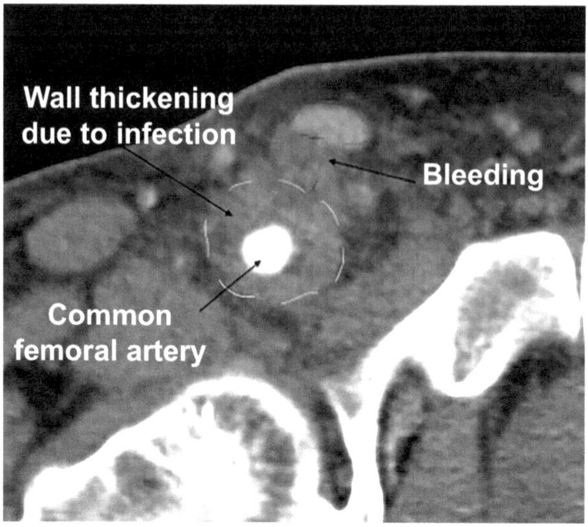

Fig. 3.1 CTA showing a septic erosion bleed in the groin after patch plasty

- less commonly popliteal
- very rarely cervical (here, patients after repeat procedures or radiation are predisposed)
- History of open or endovascular aortic procedures and recurrent fever episodes, rectal bleeding, and hematemesis (in the case of fistula formation)
- Tumor patient
  - typically patients from otorhinolaryngology (ENT)
  - with a tracheostomy in place or
  - history of radiation or neck dissection
- History of lymph node dissections for tumors with recurrences
  - groin, less commonly axilla

Typical On-Call Situation

- Often presents dramatically with acute spurting bleeding from surgical wounds or scars
- At initial examination in the emergency department, after prior compression by paramedics, bleeding has usually already stopped. But caution: after removal of the pressure dressing or inspection/manipulation of the blood clot, spurting bleeding usually recurs
- Call from endoscopy with visible bleeding source and suspected fistula between aorta or aortic prosthesis and the intestine
- Presentation from other departments, e.g., ENT for cervical skin changes after radiation or due to tracheostomy
- Groin bleeding after puncture or bypass/patch plasty

Diagnostics

- Clinical examination
  - often sufficient
  - visible pulsatile swelling or bleeding
- Laboratory
  - inflammatory markers
  - ischemia parameters (inflammation can lead to arterial thrombosis with possible additional embolization)
- Ultrasound
  - useful for superficial anastomoses to localize bleeding
  - demonstration of bypass occlusion
  - differentiation between hematoma and abscess
- CT angiography
  - fastest and most informative diagnostic tool
  - reliable identification of bleeding sources and possible abscess formation (air inclusions!)
- Angiography
  - only in readiness for intervention, not as a purely diagnostic tool
  - for embolization of peripheral eroded vessel branches or
  - for implantation of a covered stent

Therapy

- Conservative
  - Indications:
    as an initial measure
    in cases of unclear diagnosis
    if invasive therapy is declined
    inoperability and palliative treatment approach
  - Procedure:
    Compression bandage
    Pain medication
    Antibiotic therapy
    Optimization of coagulation
- Interventional
  - Indications:
    if the patient is unstable and there is active bleeding
    if technically feasible
  - Procedure:
    Embolization using coils/Onyx®
    Implantation of covered stents→ often as a bridging measure, to allow for definitive treatment after stabilization of the bleeding
- Surgical
  - Indications:
    treatment of choice in active bleeding and confirmed infectious complication

- Procedure:
  often vascular reconstruction is necessary, exclusively autologous with vein or, if necessary, xenogeneic using bovine patch material (a tubular interposition graft can also be fashioned from this)

Call the on-call service at night?

- In cases of active bleeding and hemodynamically unstable patient
- After initial cessation of bleeding and recurrence of bleeding complications on the ward

Tips and Tricks

- Even if the bleeding has completely stopped at presentation, patients should still be monitored as inpatients. The bleeding usually stops only temporarily and tends to recur
- Plastic material should be explanted and replaced autologously
- A pseudoaneurysm that has existed for a longer period after percutaneous intervention (several months/years) or only appears months later is rarely a simple puncture hole that can be easily sutured. There is usually an infection behind it and the hole is larger than expected. A simple suture is rarely sufficient; the vessel usually needs to be replaced, ideally autologously with an interposition graft
- Determine coagulation parameters and, if necessary, optimize them before surgical intervention. Patients are often on oral anticoagulants and intraoperative blood loss can be significant in situations with temporarily poor visibility!
- Ensure an adequate supply of cross-matched blood products is available

Continuation of Case Example

You order a CT angiography and prepare for surgery. The leg should be completely prepped to allow harvesting of a segment of the great saphenous vein.

Pseudoaneurysm of the Carotid Artery

4

The false aneurysm of the carotid artery is mostly iatrogenic, occurring both in connection with puncture and after carotid surgery. However, post-traumatic causes should also be considered, and clinical signs such as contusions or strangulation marks should be looked for.

Case Example
The on-call anesthesiologist from the intensive care unit contacts you after a Shaldon catheter has been removed. Following a failed puncture attempt under difficult resuscitation conditions, the catheter was apparently inserted into the common carotid artery. Now, there is massive swelling of the neck, dyspnea, and ultrasound reveals a false aneurysm of the punctured common carotid artery (Fig. 4.1). What do you recommend?

Definition
- Bleeding or pulsatile hematoma of the carotid artery

Typical Patient
- Multimorbid high-risk patient during induction of anesthesia
- Patient in the intensive care unit, typically after resuscitation
- Dialysis patient after malposition of an atrial catheter
- Patient with acute renal failure and difficult placement of a Shaldon catheter
- Status post carotid surgery
  - if recent: suspicion of technical error or suture rupture
  - if longer ago: suspicious for infection
- Post-traumatic
  - Hyperextension trauma
  - Suicide attempt by hanging
  - Violence by (manual) strangulation

S. Regus, *Vascular Surgical Emergencies*,
https://doi.org/10.1007/978-3-662-72646-4_4

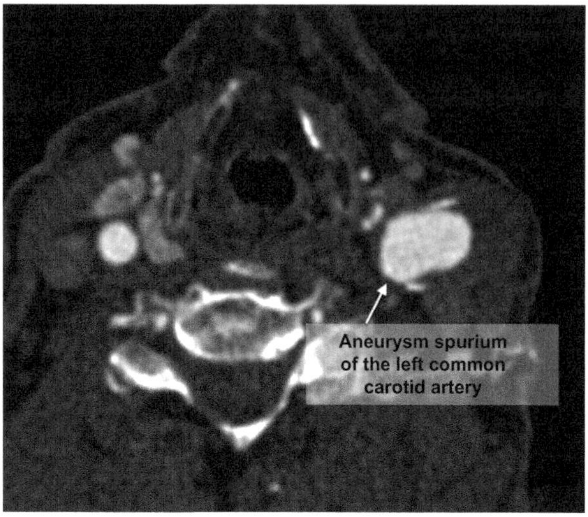

Fig. 4.1 CTA of a false aneurysm of the left common carotid artery

- Patient with oropharyngeal carcinoma
  - Status post radiation
  - existing tracheostomy and erosion

Typical On-Call Situation

- Contact from anesthesia due to cervical bleeding after puncture
- Consultation from dialysis for bleeding/pulsatile swelling of the neck
- Patient presents to the emergency department with pulsatile cervical swelling
  - sometimes present for a longer period, now painful
  - Polytrauma patient with
  - severe cervical spine trauma

Diagnostics

- Clinical examination
  - Inspection:
    - Signs of infection
      - → Redness
      - → Swelling
      - → Increased warmth
      - → Tenderness on pressure
    - Open wound
    - Visible puncture
    - Surgical scar
    - Displaced catheter
    - Auscultation
      - Bruit as an indication of an arteriovenous fistula

- Laboratory
  - Blood count (anemia, leukocytosis, thrombocytopenia?)
  - Inflammatory markers
  - Coagulation parameters
- Ultrasound
  - for orientation
  - Bleeding is usually well visualized
  - Surrounding structures are well assessable (e.g., internal jugular vein)
- CT angiography
  - Diagnostic tool of choice
  - good visualization of
    source of bleeding
    aneurysm configuration
    thrombosis above and below
    active perfusion
    cerebral bleeding or ischemia

Therapy

- Conservative
  - Indications:
    small, no longer perfused aneurysm
    no symptoms, especially no tenderness, no signs of compression
    high surgical risk due to malignant underlying disease and
    limited life expectancy
  - Approach:
    pain management
    if necessary, antibiotics in case of suspected infection
    anticoagulation in case of suspected thrombosis/embolization
    antiplatelet therapy in atherosclerosis (postoperative)
    optimization of coagulation in case of bleeding complications
- Interventional
  - Indications:
    complication with existing stent
    symptomatic aneurysm in inoperable patient, e.g., significant soft tissue scarring after multiple previous surgeries, radiation, neck dissection
  - Approach:
    implantation of a coated stent
    if necessary, embolization, though with the risk of cerebral ischemia
- Surgical
  - Indications:
    in case of active bleeding and
    signs of compression (dyspnea, dysphagia) after recent puncture or carotid surgery
    in case of catheter malposition in the artery and TIA or manifest cerebral stroke

- Approach:
  emergency revision and oversewing
  if necessary, placement of an interposition graft
  in case of catheter malposition, urgent removal and, if necessary, new placement on the contralateral side

Call the on-call service at night?

- In case of carotid complications, always call and inform. Signs of compression (trachea!) can very quickly lead to life-threatening situations.

Tips and Tricks

- Remember neuromonitoring during surgical preparation
- Visualize the great saphenous vein by ultrasound (suitable for grafting? History of great saphenous vein stripping?)
- Disinfect the leg with the better-suited great saphenous vein in a sterile manner to allow harvesting if needed
- Alternatively, use a synthetic interposition graft
- If puncture/surgery was some time ago, simple oversewing is rarely possible
- In patients with malignant underlying disease and prior cervical surgery/radiation, prefer an interventional approach, if necessary as a bridging solution

Continuation of Case Example

You arrange for emergency surgical management and have the patient taken to the OR immediately. You also recommend prompt intubation, as increasing bleeding may make this impossible in extreme cases, necessitating an emergency cricothyrotomy.

5 Pseudoaneurysm in the Groin after Puncture

The pseudoaneurysm in the groin is one of the most common acute bleeding complications that require vascular surgical expertise. It most frequently occurs after percutaneous interventions and can range from small and completely harmless to massive and life-threatening.

Case Example
Call from the ward nurse: 73-year-old female patient, underwent percutaneous transluminal angioplasty (PTA) of the right superficial femoral artery today, now experiencing massive bleeding into the right groin with hemodynamic significance, blood pressure 80 over 60, pulse 120. Clinically, there is massive swelling in the groin, patient is somnolent. What do you do? (Fig. 5.1)

Definition

- Puncture aneurysm in the groin, most commonly the common femoral artery, less frequently the profunda femoris or superficial femoral artery, or distal external iliac artery

Typical Patient

- Percutaneous intervention today or a few days ago
- Sometimes also status post intensive care treatment with arterial or venous access via the groin

Typical On-Call Situation

- Bleeding on the ward with a pressure dressing in place after percutaneous intervention
- Hemorrhagic shock in the intensive care unit due to bleeding and groin hematoma after puncture
- Patient presents to the emergency department with swelling in the groin after a recent intervention

S. Regus, *Vascular Surgical Emergencies*,
https://doi.org/10.1007/978-3-662-72646-4_5

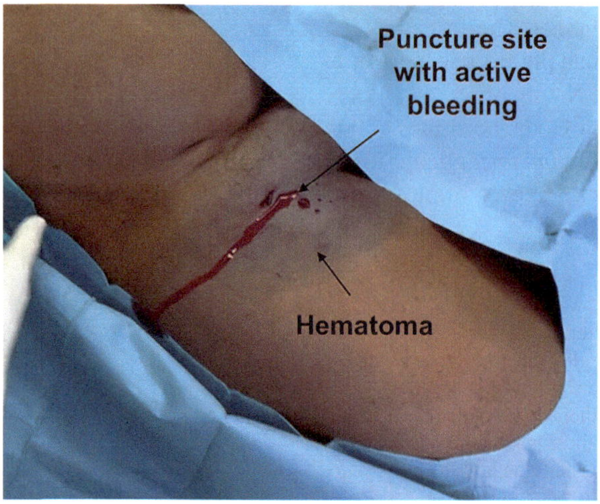

Fig. 5.1 Clinical finding of a pseudoaneurysm in the groin after puncture

Diagnostics

- Clinical examination
  - clinically, bleeding and hematoma are often already visible
  - usually a pulsatile swelling is palpable
- Laboratory tests
  - especially complete blood count (anemia?) and coagulation
- Ultrasound
  - visualization of an active bleeding source
  - vessel wall thickening
  - if the puncture was some time ago and there is suspicion of infection
  - size of the hematoma
  - active perfusion of the hematoma cavity
  - visualization of an arteriovenous fistula (if both artery and vein were injured during puncture)
- CT angiography
  - diagnostic tool of choice in hemodynamically stable patients, but only if there are therapeutic consequences due to a large hematoma requiring treatment
  - if there is only minor bleeding and stable soft tissue conditions:
    then CTA has no consequence
    initially, conservative management is indicated
  - if the patient is hemodynamically unstable and there is clear external evidence of bleeding:
    no further diagnostics, but take the patient directly to the OR

Therapy

- Conservative
  - Indications:
    small hematoma with low-grade/no longer present perfusion
    no or only mild pressure pain, soft on palpation, no skin involvement (e.g., tension blisters, livid discoloration)
  - Procedure:
    Compression bandage
    Bed rest
    Analgesic medication
    Antibiotics in case of infection
    if necessary, RBC transfusions, depending on Hb level
    Optimize coagulation
- Interventional
  - Indications:
    if conservative therapy is unsuccessful and
    ongoing perfusion as well as
    increasing pain symptoms
    Skin conditions should be unremarkable:
      no marked tension
      no tension blisters
      no suspicion of infection→ then surgery
  - Procedure:
    usually elective thrombin injection
      → performed by internists or radiologists 5000 IU thrombin in 5 ml NaCl 0.9% (1000 IU/ml) in 0.5 ml (= 500 IU) increments; usually 500–1500 IU are sufficient
    Embolization with coils
    Placement of a coated (covered) stent
- Surgical
  - Indications:
    in case of large hematoma
    in case of extensive bleeding and
    in case of compromised soft tissue conditions (tension blisters, beginning skin necrosis, etc.)
    emergency indication in hemorrhagic shock
  - Procedure:
    Suturing, hematoma evacuation, placement of a drain

Call the on-call service at night?

- If unstable, increasing in size, or bleeding that cannot be controlled by compression, then contact by phone
- If compression is successful and pain symptoms are manageable, it is sufficient to pass on the information at the morning meeting

Tips and Tricks

- Do not perform CTA in unstable patients with clear clinical findings. Time lost can cost the patient (often elderly and multimorbid) their life
- Retroperitoneal bleeding can lead to massive blood loss, even if little is visible externally
- Be cautious with patients whose puncture was some time ago: infection is often the underlying cause here, and simple suturing is rarely possible. Therefore, wash the entire leg (foot in a leg bag) to be able to harvest the great saphenous vein if necessary
- Always palpate foot pulses to avoid missing a subsequent arterial occlusion. This can typically occur due to peripheral embolization or arterial thrombosis following compression

Continuation of Case Example

You organize emergency surgical management and take the patient directly to the OR under compression of the groin. Any delay due to further diagnostics can cost the patient her life.

6 Anastomotic Aneurysm in the Groin

An anastomotic aneurysm in the groin is a common complication following patch plasty or bypass surgery with origin or insertion at the femoral bifurcation. This clinical picture is often announced acutely and dramatically, but frequently turns out to be chronic (and thus relatively harmless); however, in some cases, it can also present as a highly acute, life-threatening situation with high mortality.

Case Example

A 63-year-old unkempt patient, who had not visited his general practitioner for a long time, is admitted as an emergency by the latter. The "admission diagnosis" is aneurysm after bypass surgery. After a brief medical history, you find out that the patient underwent a right-sided iliofemoral bypass 5 years ago and has had a swelling in the groin for several months. This causes the patient no discomfort, not even currently. His walking distance has been unlimited since the bypass, and he walks into the emergency department. The surgical scars are unremarkable, and there is no discoloration. The pulsating swelling is visible to the naked eye, and there is no tenderness on pressure. Foot pulses are strong and palpable on both sides. CTA reveals an anastomotic aneurysm that has been present for some time and is well encapsulated (Fig. 6.1). Is it absolutely necessary to admit the patient as an inpatient?

Definition

- Suture insufficiency in the groin after arterial reconstruction
- Status post patch plasty or bypass surgery

Typical Patient

- Typical "vascular patient," often with multiple previous surgeries
- Reports a pulsating swelling in the groin for a long time, which is often barely or not at all painful, or

S. Regus, *Vascular Surgical Emergencies*,
https://doi.org/10.1007/978-3-662-72646-4_6

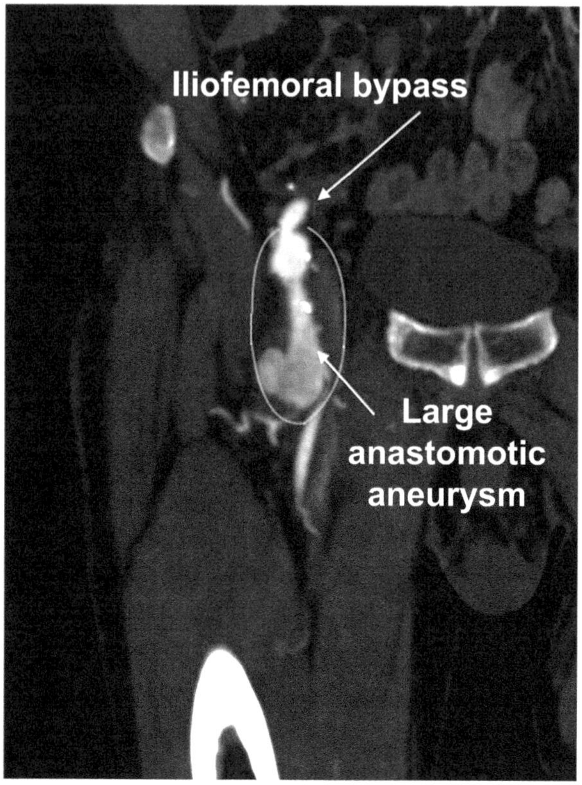

Fig. 6.1 CTA of a large anastomotic aneurysm in the groin after iliofemoral bypass surgery

- an acutely occurring painful (pressure or spontaneous pain) bulge with bleeding complication
- Sometimes also presents with infection symptoms such as redness in the groin and febrile temperatures

Typical On-Call Situation

- Patients with chronic anastomotic aneurysm usually present electively via the outpatient clinic.
- During on-call duty, most presentations are due to acute swelling with increasing pain.
- Not infrequently, there is also an "emergency" referral from the general practitioner, who is seeing the finding for the first time and wants to be on the safe side. If the patient reports that he has had this swelling for years and denies pain, diagnostics and therapy should be managed electively via the outpatient clinic.

Diagnostics

- Clinical examination
  - Scars from previous operations
  - Redness
  - Swelling
  - Tenderness on pressure
  - Fistula with secretion
- Laboratory
  - Elevated inflammatory markers: suggestive of infection
  - Elevated D-dimers: could indicate a thrombotic event
- Ultrasound
  - Aneurysm size can be determined
  - Compression of the adjacent vein visible
  - Parietal thrombi detectable (rare)
  - Signs of infection
    Wall thickening
    enlarged lymph nodes
- CT angiography
  - Extent of the aneurysm formation
  - active bleeding
  - Perfusion of inflow and outflow vessels including bypass occlusion
  - Air inclusions as a clear indication of infection

Therapy

- Conservative
  - Indications:
    small aneurysm without symptoms
    refusal of surgery
    inoperable patient due to multimorbidity
    limited life expectancy due to malignant underlying disease
  - Approach:
    pain management
    antibiotic therapy if infection is suspected
    prophylactic low-molecular-weight heparin (e.g., Clexane® 0.4 ml/40 mg) if mobility is limited, or
    therapeutic low-molecular-weight heparin (e.g., Clexane®) twice daily, weight-adjusted, if oral anticoagulation must be paused and bridging is necessary
    if necessary, Konakion® if Quick is decreased under phenprocoumon
    PPSB only in vital emergencies, as the risk of thromboembolic complications is increased

- Interventional
  - Indications:
    multiple previous surgeries or
    history of radiation therapy
  - Approach:
    placement of a coated stent (for bridging or palliative intent)
    embolization, if necessary with coils or Onyx®
- Surgical
  - Indications:
    pain
    rapid increase in size
    external and/or systemic signs of infection
    hemorrhagic shock
    sepsis
    impending disruption of skin continuity
    arterial/venous compression with ischemia
  - Approach:
    exclusion and placement of an interposition graft
    removal of synthetic patch and replacement with autologous (vein) or xenogeneic (bovine pericardium) material
    explantation of an infected bypass
    in case of irreversible ischemia, amputation ("life before limb")

Call the on-call service at night?

- If there is no active bleeding and the patient is stable, admit to the ward and keep the patient fasting for the morning rounds.
- In case of active bleeding with hemodynamic instability, urgent contact is necessary.

Tips and Tricks

- If justifiable (not a vital emergency, but urgent), postpone the surgical procedure to the next working day.
- Procedures performed on call can lead to serious complications.
- Disinfect and drape the surgical field extensively, from the nipple down to and including the leg, using sterile technique.
- If necessary, abdominal/retroperitoneal access may be required to control inflow.
- Vein harvesting may be necessary for an autologous interposition graft.
- Peripheral embolectomy/thrombectomy may be required if peripheral embolization has occurred.
- Bypass reconstruction may be necessary if ischemia is present and perfusion cannot be restored by thrombectomy.
- In case of ischemia, leave the foot exposed to assess reperfusion.

Case Example Continued

Inpatient admission is not absolutely necessary. This is clearly a chronic anastomotic aneurysm. You should rule out an arterial occlusion, which can be ensured by history (unrestricted walking distance) and pulse status (strongly palpable foot pulses). Further elective surgical planning can be organized on an outpatient basis through the clinic.

Ruptured Popliteal Aneurysm

7

The ruptured popliteal aneurysm (Fig. 7.1) is a rather rare but serious complication of a popliteal aneurysm, with a high risk (up to 50%) of limb loss. Rapid intervention is required, usually by surgical reconstruction including fasciotomy.

Case Example
A call comes in from a neighboring primary and secondary care hospital, where an 83-year-old patient has undergone a surgical procedure in the popliteal fossa: Under the presumptive diagnosis of a popliteal abscess due to marked redness and swelling, surgical abscess drainage was indicated. Intraoperatively, however, the supposed abscess turns out to be a contained rupture of a popliteal aneurysm. The colleague requests prompt transfer of the patient to vascular surgery. There is no active bleeding after adequate suturing. How do you proceed?

Definition
- Rupture and bleeding of an aneurysm of the popliteal artery
- True aneurysm usually in the context of infection (= mycotic aneurysm)
- False aneurysm post-traumatic (stab injury or knee dislocation fracture) or iatrogenic (e.g., after knee arthroplasty or arthroscopy)

Typical Patient
- Usually older patient with a cardiovascular risk profile
- Men >> women
- Not infrequently, positive "aneurysm history"
  - about every second patient has an aortic aneurysm
  - about every third patient also has a popliteal aneurysm on the other side

S. Regus, *Vascular Surgical Emergencies*,
https://doi.org/10.1007/978-3-662-72646-4_7

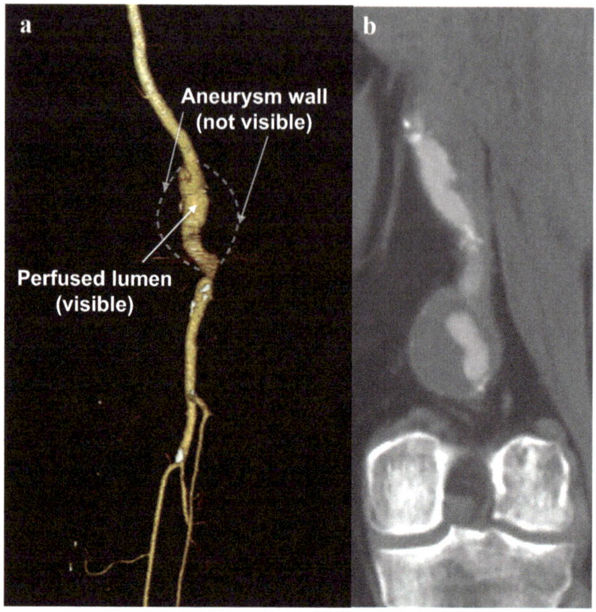

Fig. 7.1 a, b **a**MR angiographic depiction of a popliteal aneurysm, which can easily be overlooked since only the perfused lumen is visible. The aneurysm sac is not visualized due to the usually present mural thrombus.**b**In CTA, the aneurysm, aneurysm sac, and mural thrombus are visualized

- Often also peripheral ischemia due to aneurysm occlusion or embolization
- In younger patients, almost exclusively trauma or surgery (e.g., knee arthroscopy) in the medical history
  - False aneurysm

Typical On-Call Situation
- Usually via the emergency department
- Patient reports knee pain with swelling (on further questioning, this often has been present for some time)
- Sometimes also transfer from an outside hospital due to exploration of the popliteal fossa for suspected Baker's cyst, which turns out to be an aneurysm
- Consultation by internists after diagnosis of a popliteal aneurysm during infection workup and suspicion of septic spread (mycotic aneurysm)

Diagnostics
- Clinical examination
  - visible and palpable swelling/pulsation in the popliteal fossa
- Laboratory tests
  - if infection is suspected
  - blood count

- Swab (pre- or intraoperative)
- Ultrasound
  - usually only for orientation to support the presumptive diagnosis
- CT angiography
  - diagnostic method of choice
  - fast (takes only a few minutes)
  - assessment of the vessel wall, lumen, and periphery
  - also allows preliminary assessment of the great saphenous vein as a potential graft
- Do not forget histological examination of the surgical specimen to confirm or exclude vasculitis or connective tissue disease if necessary

Therapy

- Conservative
  - Indications:
    at most as a temporary measure until definitive treatment
    irreversible ischemia of the leg and the need for major amputation, which is refused (should always be documented in writing and signed!)
  - Procedure:
    Compression
    Pain medication
    Antibiotics if infection is suspected
- Interventional
  - Indications:
    if landing zones proximal and distal are >3 cm
    primarily as a bridging procedure
    →especially in suspected infection, not a permanent solution
    →suitable for temporary bleeding control and restoration of perfusion
  - Procedure:
    antegrade puncture and implantation of a covered stent (e.g., Viabahn® by Gore)
- Surgical
  - Indications:
    Bleeding
    Massive hematoma
    Ischemia
    Compartment syndrome
    Sepsis in case of infection
  - Procedure:
    usually emergency surgery
    ligation and placement of an interposition graft
    Dorsal approach
    →sometimes limited visibility
    →extension of the procedure proximally and distally can be difficult

Medial approach in supine position
→approach of choice
→best visibility
→extension proximally and distally possible
→harvesting of the great saphenous vein possible

Call the on-call service at night?

- Usually an emergency indication and contact is necessary

Tips and Tricks

- Prefer surgery in the supine position whenever possible, as access can be easily extended proximally and distally
- In case of doubt, opt for alloplastic reconstruction, especially if there is time pressure due to ischemia
- Take a swab intraoperatively (infection?)
- Do not forget histological examination of the surgical specimen! (Inflammation? Arteriosclerosis? Connective tissue disease?)

Continuation of Case Example

Of course, you are prepared to take over the patient and ask your colleague to apply a pressure bandage to the patient and administer 5000 IU heparin as a bolus. The colleague, surprised, asks whether he should really give heparin in the event of a bleeding complication, which you confirm once again. You fear that the sufficiently tight suture (the bleeding had stopped) could lead to arterial occlusion and want to prevent progression. You inform your on-call service, OR nursing staff, anesthesia, and emergency department about the patient and the emergency surgical indication.

Part III
Arterial Occlusions

Acute Arterial Occlusion of the Leg

8

The "acute occlusion," also referred to in clinical jargon as the "cold leg," is one of the most important emergencies in vascular surgery and the most common surgical indication outside of regular working hours (Fig. 8.1).

Case Study
An 84-year-old female patient is admitted with the suspected diagnosis of an arterial occlusion. She comes from assisted living, is spry, and reports that for the past 2 hours she has suddenly had a cold foot and can no longer feel it properly. She had no complaints prior to this. On clinical examination, you already detect a weakened groin pulse on the affected side, while on the opposite side the pulses are strong down to the foot, although arrhythmic. Sonography reveals an embolus at the right femoral bifurcation. Should you order a CTA?

Definition
- Acute onset occlusion of an extremity artery
- Lower > upper extremity (approx. 20:1)
- Up to 14 days after symptom onset; after that, it is referred to as chronic circulatory disorder in the sense of peripheral arterial occlusive disease

Classification
- according to Rutherford/TASC (Trans Atlantic InterSociety Consensus)
  - I: compensated, sensorimotor function intact, pain on exertion, elective treatment possible,
    but note: By definition, acute ischemia is present only within the first 14 days; from day 15 onward, it is more correctly classified as PAOD stage II according to Fontaine
  - IIa: moderately compensated, sensation impaired, motor function intact, treatment within 24–48 h

S. Regus, *Vascular Surgical Emergencies*,
https://doi.org/10.1007/978-3-662-72646-4_8

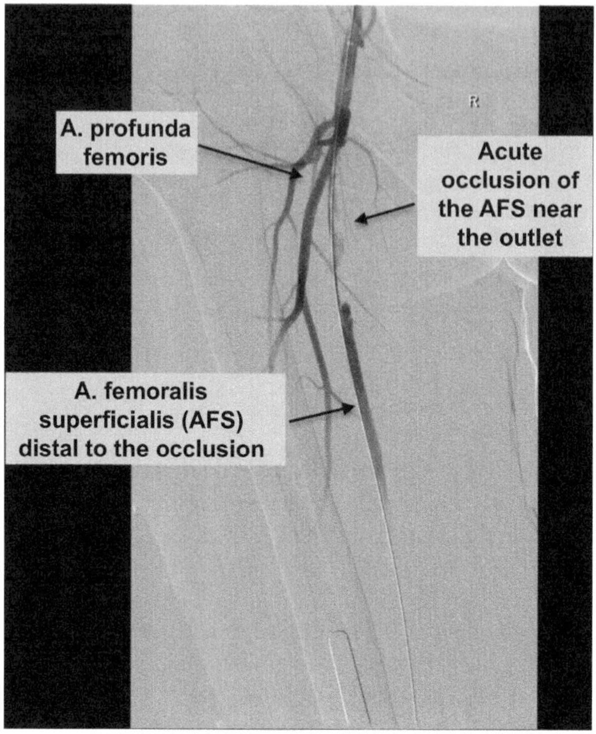

Fig. 8.1 Angiographic image of an acute occlusion of the right superficial femoral artery

- IIb: not compensated, sensorimotor function impaired, revascularization indicated within 6 h
- III: decompensated, sensorimotor function completely lost, limb not salvageable, amputation indicated

Typical Patient

- Older patient with corresponding cardiovascular risk profile (CAD, arterial hypertension, diabetes mellitus, nicotine abuse)
- Known and previous surgical as well as interventional vascular reconstructions
- Sometimes also "vascularly healthy" in cases of embolism and atrial fibrillation
- Not infrequently, the patient has a pacemaker

Typical On-Call Situation

- Notification of a "cold leg" by emergency services
- Consultation from other wards with the suspected diagnosis of an arterial occlusion

- Typical risk constellation after percutaneous intervention (neurology, neuroradiology, cardiology, radiology)
  - here, often arterial thrombosis in the groin
  - possibly with peripheral embolization (popliteal artery!)
  - sometimes also caused by incorrectly placed closure device
- Classically, in a patient with hypovolemic or cardiogenic shock and pre-existing PAOD

Case example: 55-year-old intubated smoker with a myocardial infarction who developed a cold, lividly discolored left foot while in cardiogenic shock. The coronary intervention was performed via the brachial artery. CTA shows a short-segment occlusion of the common iliac artery on the affected side, and the anesthesia colleagues request a vascular surgery consult for "acute pelvic occlusion." However, after successful resuscitation and restoration of adequate circulation, the finding completely resolves. After extubation, the patient reports that he had previously had severe claudication symptoms on the right side and could only walk 50–100 meters. In this case, it is best not to indicate invasive or surgical therapy, but simply to wait and "keep cool." Excessive interventionism can cause harm.

- Pulseless and livid leg in non-communicative, demented patients from nursing homes
  - often Rutherford III and amputation indicated

Diagnostics

- Clinical examination
  - Signs of ischemia = 5 Ps according to Pratt
    - Pulse status (Pulselessness)
    - Paleness
    - Pain
    - Paresthesia (Sensory loss)
    - Paralysis (Motor function)
      - *Note:* The "6th P according to Pratt" (Prostration = shock) has been deliberately omitted, as it is rarely used or seen in clinical practice.
  - Determination of the ankle-brachial Doppler index (Ankle Brachial Index, ABI)
- Laboratory
  - Creatine kinase (CK), myoglobin
  - Coagulation
- Sonography
  - Sufficient in cases with clear findings
    - Embolus in the femoral bifurcation or popliteal artery is well visualized
    - Arrhythmic patient
    - Foot pulses palpable on the contralateral side

No significant signs of arteriosclerosis

→then, without further diagnostics, immediate therapy indication should be established

- CT angiography
  - Diagnostic tool of choice in complex or unclear cases

    Rapidly available

    Highly informative

    Generally recommended in suspected arterial thrombosis and vessels previously damaged by atherosclerosis (not in embolism with healthy vessels)

    Indicators for arterial thrombosis are:

    →Previous surgeries (bypasses)

    →Patient is in sinus rhythm

    →Calcifications visible on sonography

    →No pulses palpable on the contralateral side

Therapy

- Conservative
  - Indications:

    Mild or asymptomatic occlusion

    Inoperable patient

    Refusal of surgical intervention

    Irreversible ischemia (Rutherford III)
  - Approach:

    Pain management

    Antiplatelet therapy and/or

    Anticoagulation

    For Rutherford I ischemia: close monitoring

    For Rutherford III ischemia: depending on treatment preferences

    →If amputation is refused and the family wishes, palliative care until end of life (usually a few days) can also be provided at home

    →However, it is important to document in writing that amputation is being refused!

Example of a common scenario: a 92-year-old demented female patient with chronic atrial fibrillation without anticoagulation due to recurrent cerebral hemorrhages presents to the emergency department. She comes from a nursing home and has a lividly discolored leg, which is cold and shows complete loss of sensorimotor function. The patient is unable to express her wishes, her daughter is the legal guardian and, in accordance with her mother's presumed wishes, refuses above-knee amputation. This is in principle reasonable and entirely justifiable, but it is important to document the refusal of amputation in writing. Only in this way can treating physicians protect themselves against potential lawsuits and claims for damages.

- Interventional
  - Indications:
    In stage IIa according to Rutherford
    If treatment is desired and there is significant suffering, also in stage I
    For short-segment stenoses/occlusions
    Crural occlusions, even if longer, are often treated interventionally
  - Approach:
    Lysis therapy
    Percutaneous transluminal angioplasty (PTA)
    Stent implantation
    CERAB ("covered endovascular repair of aortic bifurcation")
- Surgical
  - Indications:
    Stage IIb with time pressure
    Aortic occlusions extending up to the renal arteries
    After unsuccessful endovascular approach
    For Rutherford III ischemia and treatment request (amputation)
    Compartment syndrome (fasciotomy)
  - Approach:
    Embolectomy for embolic occlusion (in soft vessels, transverse arteriotomy)
    Thrombectomy with patch for arterial thrombosis
    Bypass surgery if revascularization is unsuccessful
    Major amputation
    Fasciotomy

Call the on-call service at night?
- Depending on the stage of ischemia
- In the stage of critical acute ischemia (Rutherford IIb), always call and perform emergency surgery
- For Rutherford I, IIa, or even III, information on the following day is sufficient, but keep patients fasting for the ward round

Tips and Tricks
- Always palpate pulses on the contralateral side
- If present, then embolism is likely
- If no pulses are palpable on the contralateral side and ABI is reduced, there is a suspicion of PAD
- Administer heparin at the time of diagnosis, usually as a 5000 IU bolus, often already given by the emergency physician. Therefore, inquire at handover or check the protocol
- Postoperatively, be critical when indicating a heparin infusion, as this increases the risk of bleeding and there is no proven benefit regarding bypass patency.

The surgeon decides. Especially with additional fasciotomy, significant blood loss through the large wound area may occur under heparin administration

- Indicate and perform fasciotomy generously. Better too early than too late! No patient complains about additional incisions on the leg, which usually heal well. The most common reason for patient complaints is limb loss

Continuation of Case Example

You do not need to perform a CTA for this patient (of course depending on and in consideration of internal hospital standards), but can make the diagnosis of an embolic occlusion based solely on the clinical findings (arrhythmia, strong palpable foot pulses on the contralateral side, sonographically confirmed embolus in the femoral bifurcation) and prepare the patient for surgical intervention. This should be performed as soon as possible, and at the latest within 6 hours.

Peripheral Arterial Occlusive Disease (PAOD) Stage IV

9

"Black toes" are, so to speak, part of everyday life in vascular surgery (Fig. 9.1). They are also encountered very frequently while on duty, so knowledge of diagnostics and therapy is essential.

Case Study
A 79-year-old patient, diabetic with poorly controlled blood sugar (HbA1c 11.1%), is brought to the emergency department. His wife reports that he has had a black toe for several days and has also had a fever since the previous day. In addition, he has already had his "arteries" dilated several times. On examination, you see a wet gangrene of the right big toe with redness of the entire forefoot, temperature is elevated to 38.9°C, and the patient appears severely compromised. The ankle-brachial index (ABI) on the affected side is reduced to 0.3, a femoral pulse is palpable, but popliteal and foot pulses are not palpable. Sonographically, there is suspicion of a long-segment occlusion of the superficial femoral artery. Do you prepare the patient for an MRA and bypass surgery including toe amputation the following day?

Definition

- ≥14 days of persistent arterial occlusion in the lower extremity with trophic skin lesions

Classification

- According to Fontaine, stages I–IV
  - I: asymptomatic
  - II: pain on exertion
  - III: pain at rest
  - IV: trophic skin lesions

S. Regus, *Vascular Surgical Emergencies*,
https://doi.org/10.1007/978-3-662-72646-4_9

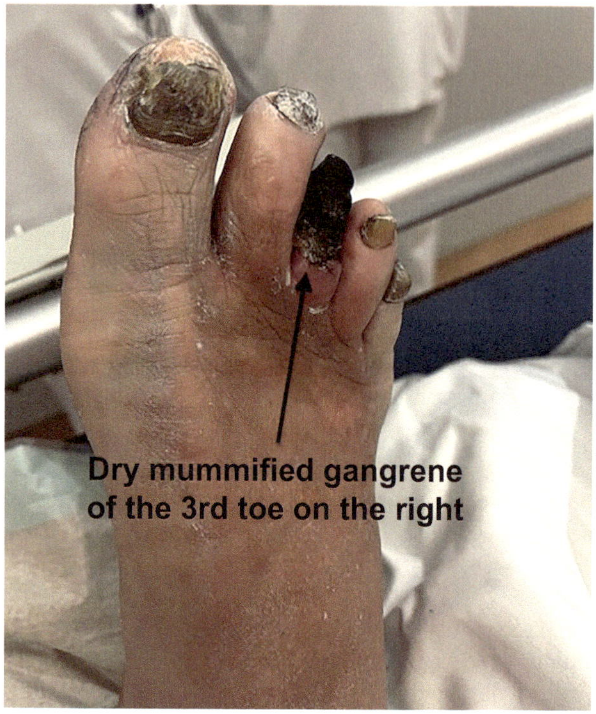

Fig. 9.1 Clinical finding of PAD stage IV with dry gangrene of the third toe on the right

- According to Rutherford, stages 0–6
  - 0: asymptomatic
  - 1: mild pain on exertion
  - 2: moderate pain on exertion
  - 3: severe pain on exertion
  - 4: pain at rest
  - 5: superficial ulcers
  - 6: deep ulcers

Typical Patient
- Patient with chronic ulcer on the lower leg (lateral >> medial)
- Black toes for a longer period, now with increasing pain, redness, putrid discharge, and fever
- Known PAD, previous peripheral surgeries and interventions
- Long-standing diabetic with advanced ulcers and soft tissue infections
- Often already status post toe amputations or major contralateral amputation

Typical On-Call Situation

- Presentation to the emergency department with fever, chills, increasing pain
- Often also patients from nursing homes with "black foot," frequently on Friday evenings or before holidays (Christmas/Easter)
- Consultation from dialysis for black toes for further evaluation
- Patient from cardiology with known or suspected PAD (comorbidity!) for further evaluation and possible transfer

Diagnostics

- Clinical examination
  - acral ulcers and gangrene, nonviable, often with exposed tendons or joints
  - ulcers lateral and on the dorsum of the foot (medial suggests venous etiology)
  - foot pulses not palpable
  - ABI often reduced to ≤ 0.5
- Ultrasound
  - stenoses/occlusions
  - monophasic signals often already detectable in the popliteal fossa
- X-ray in 2 planes
  - osteolyses
  - dislocations
- MRA
  - for therapy planning
- Digital subtraction angiography (DSA)
  - antegrade if intervention is planned, when femoral, popliteal, or crural stenoses are suspected
  - retrograde or crossover for iliac stenotic processes

Therapy

- Conservative
  - Indications:
    for superficial ulcers and
    exclusion of hemodynamically significant stenoses
    when the patient is immobile/bedridden/with contractures in the hip and knee joints
    → elaborate bypass reconstructions are not justified
    → DSA/percutaneous transluminal angioplasty (PTA) in some cases only possible under anesthesia (in cases of dementia/noncompliance) with a high risk of postoperative bleeding
    → Major ablation should be postponed as long as possible in the case of superficial ulcers
  - Procedure:
    Wound cleansing
    preferably dry dressings
    Cotton padding

Antibiotic therapy in case of infection (use with caution)
Pain management

- Interventional
  - Indications:
    short-segment stenoses/occlusions
    bypass occlusion
    stent occlusion
    in-stent stenosis
  - Procedure:
    Angiography with readiness for intervention
    PTA/stent
    Lysis
    Aspiration thrombectomy
- Surgical
  - Indications:
    long-segment occlusions
    unsuccessful interventional attempt
    deep soft tissue infections
    extensive gangrene/ulcers
    non-salvageable limb
  - Procedure:
    surgical bypass reconstruction
    wound debridement, if necessary with VAC® system
    amputation

Call the on-call service at night?

- Usually not necessary, information on the following day is sufficient
- Keep the patient fasting for the ward round in case surgery needs to be performed

Tips and Tricks

- In toe gangrene without significant signs of infection and short-segment arterial stenoses
  - initially interventional recanalization
  - then amputation
- In toe gangrene without significant signs of infection and long-segment stenoses/occlusions
  - surgical vascular reconstruction and toe amputation early-electively (not as an emergency) in a "single session"
- In toe gangrene with local and systemic signs of infection
  - urgent indication for toe amputation/abscess drainage/debridement
  - then earliest possible elective vascular reconstruction

- No elaborate reconstruction in non-salvageable limb
  - may lead to septic "showering"
- If possible, do not debride a dry heel necrosis in bedridden patients treated conservatively
  - debridement can turn a stable condition into an unstable one with sepsis, bleeding complications, and a finding requiring amputation

Continuation of Case Example

Since the patient clearly presents with a pronounced infectious constellation with systemic dissemination, toe amputation should be performed on the day of admission. Ideally, a regional anesthesia technique is possible for this. Subsequently, however, surgical bypass placement is indicated as soon as possible, ideally on the following day and after prior imaging with MRA. Only in this way is undisturbed wound healing possible.

Acute Arterial Occlusion of the Arm 10

In clinical jargon, "acute occlusion" of the arm is referred to as a "cold arm" and is a typical, but much less common, emergency than acute occlusion of a leg artery. Almost without exception, it is caused by an arterial embolism with the embolic source being the "heart," such as in atrial fibrillation or a ventricular aneurysm (Fig. 10.1).

Case Study

A 42-year-old obese patient complains of a cold sensation in his left arm for about 2 hours. Previously, he occasionally experienced tingling in his fingers, which, however, always resolved quickly. He takes acetylsalicylic acid 100 mg once daily due to a history of myocardial infarction 3 years ago. Vascular diseases are known in his family. On clinical examination, both the brachial and wrist pulses are absent on the affected side. On the opposite side, these pulses are strong and regular. Sonography reveals a thrombotic occlusion of the brachial artery. Based on your findings, would you take the patient to the OR with the suspected diagnosis of left brachial artery occlusion without further diagnostics?

Definition

- Acute occlusion of a shoulder-arm artery, usually the brachial (cubital) artery including the bifurcation
- "Cold" arm

Typical Patient

- Usually older patient with known cardiac arrhythmias
- Often on oral anticoagulation
  - poorly controlled (Marcumar® and Quick >40%)
  - paused due to another surgery (e.g., dental surgery)
- Occasionally also younger patients with a dialysis shunt

S. Regus, *Vascular Surgical Emergencies*,
https://doi.org/10.1007/978-3-662-72646-4_10

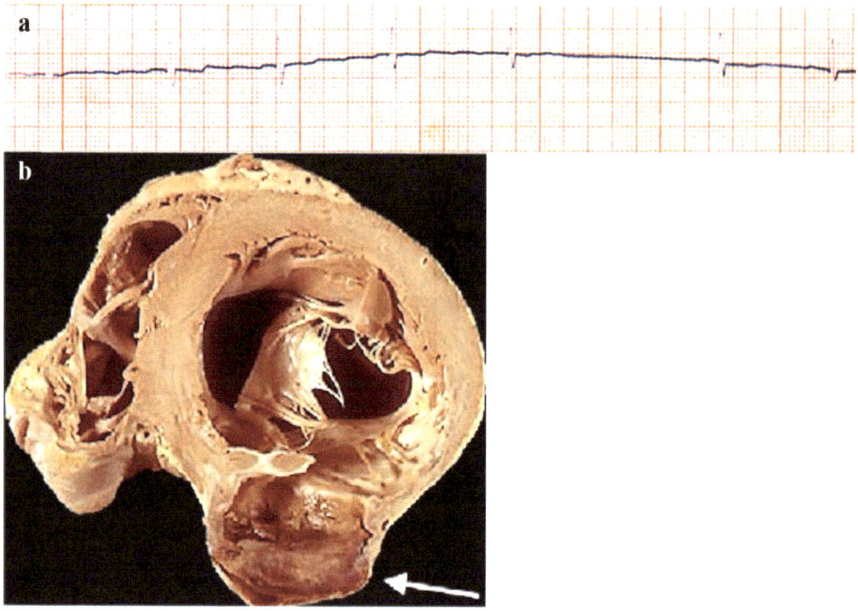

Fig. 10.1 a, b **a** Typical ECG in a patient with chronic arrhythmia due to atrial fibrillation and an embolic occlusion,**b** Ventricular aneurysm after posterior wall infarction with intracardiac thrombus (arrow) as the embolic source

- Rarely trauma-related, e.g., with shoulder dislocation and avulsion or dissection of the axillary artery
- Even more rarely sports-associated, e.g., in thoracic outlet syndrome (TOS)

Typical On-Call Situation

- Presentation to the emergency department with a "cold hand" or
- Consultation from neurology or cardiology
- Not infrequently, patients are initially admitted due to embolic stroke or suspected myocardial infarction with pain radiating into the arm, and are then subsequently referred to vascular surgery. These consultation requests often occur outside of regular working hours.

Diagnostics

- Clinical examination
  - cold hand
  - livid discoloration

    rare, as collateral circulation is usually good
  - no palpable pulses at the wrist
  - possibly a percussion pulse palpable in the antecubital fossa
  - if the embolus is lodged just below the brachial bifurcation
  - pulse often arrhythmic

- Laboratory
  - Coagulation
    often the first indication of poorly controlled oral anticoagulants
  - Blood count
    thrombocytosis?
- Sonography
  - B-mode already visualizes the hypoechoic embolus
- ECG
  - to confirm and classify a cardiac arrhythmia
  - often atrial fibrillation
  - long-term ECG may be indicated in the course
- Echocardiography
  - Detection or exclusion of an intracardiac thrombus
  - if ventricular aneurysm is suspected
    in particular, this should be ruled out after myocardial infarction
  - in valvular heart disease
    septic embolization possible
- CT angiography
  - in exceptional cases
    e.g., if aortic occlusion is suspected or
    additionally cerebral or vertebrobasilar embolization
    after trauma
    in "atypical" patients: regular rhythm, younger
      → it could also be an aneurysm of the supplying arteries or
      → an aortic dissection could be the underlying cause

Therapy

- Conservative
  - Indications:
    if asymptomatic occlusion
    compensated occlusion and elective surgery possible
    in inoperable patients
  - Procedure:
    Heparin as a bolus (5000 IU)
    Heparin infusion pump (1000 IU/24 h, target aPTT 60–80) or
    weight-adjusted low-molecular-weight heparin (e.g., enoxaparin = Clexane® 2 × daily mg per kg body weight)
    if necessary, unfractionated heparin s.c. (e.g., heparin = Liquemin® 5000 IU 3 × daily)
    Pain medication
- Interventional
  - Indications (very rare):
    in short-segment occlusion
    in patients with previous surgery or
    in patients with prior radiation
    in simultaneous cerebral occlusion

- Procedure:
  Systemic or local thrombolysis
  if necessary, with percutaneous transluminal angioplasty (PTA)
- Surgical
  - Indications:
    with few exceptions, every clearly embolic occlusion of the brachial bifurcation is an indication for surgery
    in pronounced ischemia
    in compartment syndrome
  - Procedure:
    Embolectomy, also possible under local anesthesia
    with fasciotomy (rarely necessary)

Call the on-call service at night?
- Usually not necessary in compensated ischemia, information on the following day is sufficient
  - but depends on internal departmental standards!
  - In any case, keep the patient fasting for rounds to allow for possible surgery
- In decompensated ischemia, emergency surgery must be performed and contact is essential

Tips and Tricks
- Due to good collateralization, the clinical findings are often well compensated
- Nevertheless, after confirmation of diagnosis, surgical embolectomy should be performed as soon as possible
- Postoperatively, there is often an indication for oral anticoagulation
- NOAC (e.g., rivaroxaban = Xarelto® 20 mg once daily) or
- Oral anticoagulation (phenprocoumon = Marcumar® according to INR/Quick)

Case Study Continuation
In this case, a CT angiography of the supraaortic branches including the axillary artery is definitely recommended. The patient case is not a typical and seemingly "simple" constellation; from a differential diagnostic perspective, given the age and history, an embolic process in the supplying branches (stenosis, plaque rupture, or an aneurysm) could also be causative. To avoid intraoperative surprises, it is therefore essential in such cases to perform cross-sectional imaging.

Part IV
Venous Occlusions

Thrombophlebitis of the Arm Veins 11

Thrombophlebitis of the arm is in most cases due to a peripheral venous access, making it a common reason for consultation and a frequent complication on the ward. It is generally harmless and can be treated conservatively. In cases of recurrent thrombophlebitis without an obvious cause, malignancy should be ruled out (keyword: migratory/saltatory thrombophlebitis).

Case Example

A 53-year-old female patient who received intravenous antibiotic therapy for a lobar pneumonia presents with thrombophlebitis of the median cubital vein while the cannula is still in place (Fig. 11.1). Sonography also reveals an intraluminal thrombus approximately 3 cm in length. Does the patient require oral anticoagulation?

Definition

- Short-segment thrombosis of a superficial vein with accompanying inflammation of the venous wall
- Most commonly in the antecubital fossa, forearm, and hand; rarely in the upper arm

Typical Patient

- Patient with peripheral venous access
  - may have been placed several days or weeks prior, so history is important
- In younger patients, sometimes a history of recurrent thrombophlebitis in the arms
  - Migratory/saltatory thrombophlebitis as a differential diagnosis
  - consider neoplasia in these cases, but always phrase cautiously!
- Not infrequently, known (or as yet undiagnosed) thrombophilia

S. Regus, *Vascular Surgical Emergencies*,
https://doi.org/10.1007/978-3-662-72646-4_11

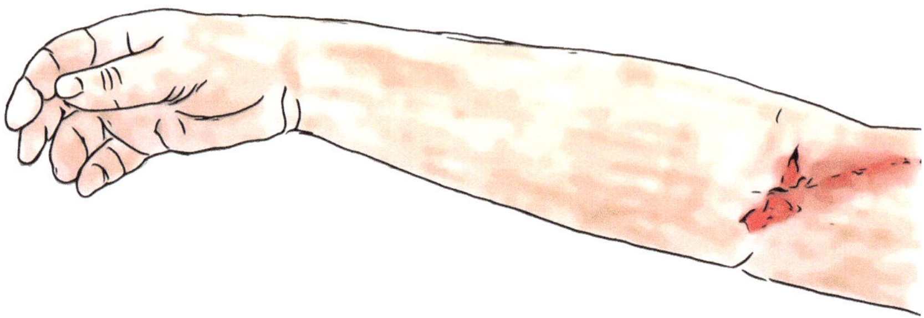

Fig. 11.1 Schematic representation of the clinical finding of thrombophlebitis in the area of the antecubital fossa following placement of a peripheral intravenous cannula

Typical On-Call Situation

- Inpatient with an indwelling cannula and a painful, reddened cord
- Presentation to the emergency department with similar symptoms, usually following recent infusion therapy

Diagnostics

- Clinical examination
  - usually a visual diagnosis
- Laboratory tests
  - usually unnecessary and without consequence
- Sonography
  - thrombus
  - thickened venous wall
- Further diagnostics are rarely indicated

Therapy

- Conservative
  - Indications:
    in cases with mild and regressing findings
    possible and indicated in the vast majority of cases
  - Procedure:
    Remove the cannula!
    Switch medication to oral administration if possible, or discontinue

oral pain management
if access is still needed, place a new one contralaterally or insert a central venous catheter
anti-inflammatory ointments
if necessary, heparin ointment
cooling
elastic compression bandaging (as tolerated)
Anticoagulation usually not necessary
→only in cases of progressive findings
→if the deep venous system is involved
→**Fondaparinux (Arixtra®)** prophylactically 2.5mg once daily or therapeutically 7.5mg once daily

- Surgical
  - Indications:
    in cases of marked swelling and redness over the thrombus
    worsening despite conservative measures
  - Procedure:
    Expressing the thrombus through a small incision
    antiseptic dressings

Call the on-call consultant at night?
- Usually not necessary, information the following day is sufficient

Tips and Tricks
- Conservative treatment is usually possible
- Anticoagulation is only rarely indicated (e.g., if the deep venous system is involved)
- Antibiotic therapy is only necessary in cases with pronounced findings
- Consider paraneoplasia if there is no clearly identifiable cause, or
- in cases with changing localization (saltatory or migratory thrombophlebitis), also consider an as yet undiagnosed tumor (e.g., testicular tumor in young men) or autoimmune diseases. Further evaluation should be initiated or at least recommended.

Continuation of Case Study
Oral anticoagulation is generally not necessary. It is sufficient to remove the cannula, cool the inflamed area, and treat it with analgesic ointments. Under these measures, the findings usually resolve completely within 1–2 weeks. Antibiotic therapy is only necessary in exceptional cases.

12 Deep Vein Thrombosis of the Leg

Most thromboses affect the deep veins of the leg below the inguinal ligament, are ascending, and are almost always treatable conservatively. Ascending pelvic vein thromboses in young women (keywords: May-Thurner syndrome–smoking–"the pill"), on the other hand, are an indication for surgery (Fig. 12.1).

Case Example
A 32-year-old pregnant woman (30th week of pregnancy) is referred to you from the gynecological outpatient clinic. She has noticed swelling of her left leg for several days, the symptoms are progressive, and there is suspicion of thrombosis. Sonography reveals a three-level venous thrombosis with the proximal end at the level of the superficial femoral vein. What do you recommend?

Definition
- Abbreviation: DVT
- Clot formation in the deep veins of the leg (also called major veins)
- Usually ascending = starting distally and progressing proximally
- Rarely descending = "descending" from proximal to distal
- Superficial veins may be partially involved, but if isolated, these thromboses are called thrombophlebitis.

Typical Patient
- Younger women (20–45 years)
- Nicotine abuse and "the pill"
- History of air/bus/car travel with limited mobility
- Recent surgical procedure, usually on the lower extremity, classic example: knee arthroscopy

S. Regus, *Vascular Surgical Emergencies*,
https://doi.org/10.1007/978-3-662-72646-4_12

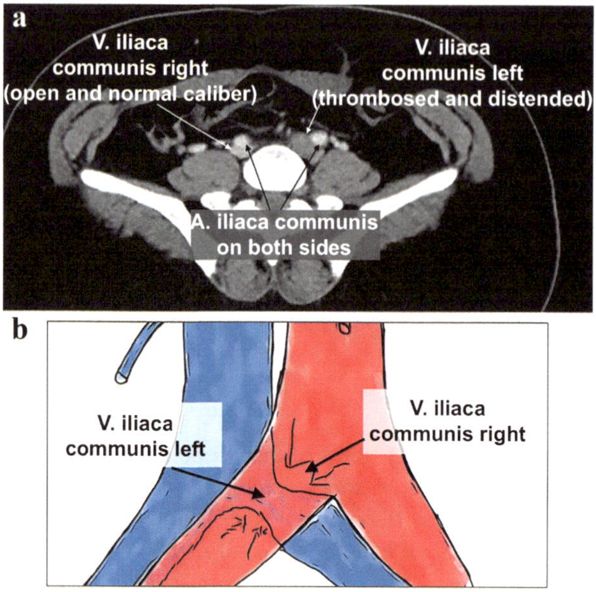

Fig. 12.1 a, b **a** CT angiographic depiction of a thrombosis of the left common iliac vein in a young woman with May-Thurner syndrome, **b** schematic illustration of May-Thurner syndrome with compression of the left common iliac vein by the right common iliac artery

- History of thrombosis or positive family history
- Rare, but not to be underestimated: long-distance runners are also at risk of developing a leg vein thrombosis after prolonged exertion and dehydration (training, competition).

Typical Situation on Duty
- Leg swelling for a few days, initial evaluation by general practitioner, then admission with suspected diagnosis of "DVT"
- Consultation request for an inpatient with leg swelling
- In some cases, patients in the intensive care unit without leg swelling, but with suspected or confirmed pulmonary embolism
- Thrombophlebitis of the great saphenous vein with suspected involvement of the deep venous system

Diagnostics
- History and clinical examination
  - Assess Wells score (this should be available as a table in the emergency department). You can remember that the score includes
  - 5 questions on history:
    positive *personal* history

  positive *family* history
  recent prolonged *travel*
  recent *surgical* procedure
  known *malignancy* and
  - 5 questions on findings
    edematous *swelling*
    difference in circumference
    visible *vein pattern*
    tenderness along the course of the vein
    visible *varicose veins*
  - A positive finding scores 1 point each
  - If an alternative differential diagnosis is present, subtract 2 points
  - Wells score
    < 2: Thrombosis unlikely
    2 or more: Thrombosis likely, sonography recommended
- Laboratory
  - no routine laboratory testing necessary
  - in particular, no routine determination of D-dimers. The latter are nonspecific and do not prove thrombosis
  - only if D-dimers are negative and Wells score < 2 can they help the clinician, as thrombosis can then be ruled out with high probability and sonography can be omitted

- Sonography
  - Compression sonography
  - "Two-point sonography" in the groin (including respiratory modulation) and popliteal fossa
  - fast and informative
  - more difficult and highly examiner-dependent in the lower leg

- CT phlebography
  - "CTA with venous phase"
  - if there is suspicion of central extension

- CT thorax
  - in case of dyspnea with "pulmonary phase"
  - to rule out pulmonary embolism

Therapy
- Conservative
  - Indications:
    possible in > 90% of cases
    ascending TBVT and swelling and pain manageable conservatively
      → rule out phlegmasia coerulea dolens
    upper limit below the inguinal ligament

→ rule out isolated pelvic vein thrombosis and
→ no involvement of the vena cava
cardiorespiratorily stable patient
→ rule out pulmonary embolism
- Procedure:
Anticoagulation
→ unfractionated heparin (only for inpatient treatment)
Start infusion rate at 2 ml/h (=1000 IU/h)
→ weight-adjusted low-molecular-weight heparin 2×daily (e.g., Enoxaparin = Clexane®) or
→ NOAC (e.g., Rivaroxaban = Xarelto®: 15 mg 2×daily for 3 weeks, from week 4: 20 mg 1×daily) or
→ oral anticoagulation with phenprocoumon (Marcumar®), 3–2–1, then coagulation monitoring, target INR 2–3 (-Quick 20–30%)
→ duration 3–6 months, then re-evaluation
Compression therapy
→ initially wrap with elastic compression and mobilize
→ after swelling subsides, fit a medical compression stocking
→ standard is class II (=MKS Ccl 2), A–G ("thigh-high stocking") or A–D ("knee-high stocking")

- Interventional
  - Indications:
    4-level venous thrombosis in young women
    pelvic vein spur (May-Thurner syndrome)
    recurrent occlusion
    chronic outflow problem
  - Procedure:
    lysis therapy
    percutaneous transluminal angioplasty (PTA)/stent implantation if an obstruction is detected
- Surgical
  - Indications: **There are two urgent or emergency surgical indications that should be known:**
    Isolated pelvic vein thrombosis, especially in young women (May-Thurner syndrome), and
    Phlegmasia coerulea dolens, in which complete interruption of venous outflow leads to soft tissue swelling. If tissue pressure continues to increase, in addition to the venous outflow problem, there is also impairment of arterial inflow, which then constitutes an emergency indication for surgical intervention, including, in some cases, compartment splitting.
  - Procedure:
    open thrombectomy via the groin
    → centrally using a Fogarty catheter
    → peripherally manually by "milking" or "expressing"
    → if necessary, stent implantation in the pelvis

→ if necessary, AV fistula in the groin to increase flow and minimize immediate or early risk of occlusion
→ fasciotomy of the lower leg

Call the on-call service at night?

- Usually not necessary, information the following day is sufficient
- Keep the patient fasting for rounds in case surgery needs to be performed

Tips and Tricks

- Fitting a medical compression stocking should always be done in the morning after swelling has subsided (outpatients often ask about this)
- In case of dyspnea, do not forget CT thorax with "pulmonary phase" (it is best to call the radiologists yourself and request this)
- For uncomplicated thromboses, ultrasound follow-up after 3–6 months
- In case of recurrence, thrombophilia screening is recommended after completion of anticoagulation
- Phlegmasia coerulea dolens is extremely rare; a "livid, swollen" leg is not proof
  - Most important criterion: arterial perfusion
  - Palpable foot pulses rule out manifest phlegmasia coerulea dolens
- Phlegmasia coerulea dolens is often a sign of a serious underlying condition (malignancy, severe thrombophilia, hematological disorder)
- May-Thurner syndrome
  - is pronounced as written, i.e., "Mai-Turner," since May was a German vascular surgeon and Thurner a pathologist from Austria
  - describes a left pelvic vein spur due to the crossing of the left common iliac vein beneath the right common iliac artery

Continuation of Case Example

It is also important to know whether the patient has dyspnea (she does not) and whether this is the first event (she has not had a thrombosis before). Then you recommend compression therapy and administration of a low-molecular-weight heparin in therapeutic dosage (2×daily, weight-adjusted). Oral anticoagulants, both phenprocoumon and NOACs, are contraindicated during pregnancy.

Thrombosis of the Axillary/Arm Veins

13

Conservative therapy using compression and anticoagulation forms the basis of treatment measures for arm vein thrombosis, as long as no direct trigger is identifiable. In the case of foreign bodies (usually port catheters), explantation should be pursued as soon as this is possible given the underlying disease.

Case Example

A 67-year-old female patient has a port catheter on the right side, through which she is receiving chemotherapy for breast cancer on the left side. The chemotherapy is nearly complete, the port is functioning without problems, and both clinically and sonographically she has a fresh thrombosis of the right subclavian vein with an unremarkably compressible internal jugular vein (Fig. 13.1). The attending gynecologists ask whether the port catheter must be removed immediately. What do you recommend?

Definition

- Thrombosis of the deep veins of the arm/shoulder
- After physical exertion/sports also referred to as "effort thrombosis"
- Synonym: Paget-von-Schroetter syndrome

Typical Patient

- Younger, athletic men
- Most often right side
- Muscular patients (bodybuilders, rowers, climbers)

Typical Situation on Duty

- Presentation to the emergency department due to arm swelling
- Occasionally also shortness of breath (rare)
- More common in summer (dehydration)
- Typically after sports or competition
- Not a life-threatening situation

S. Regus, *Vascular Surgical Emergencies*,
https://doi.org/10.1007/978-3-662-72646-4_13

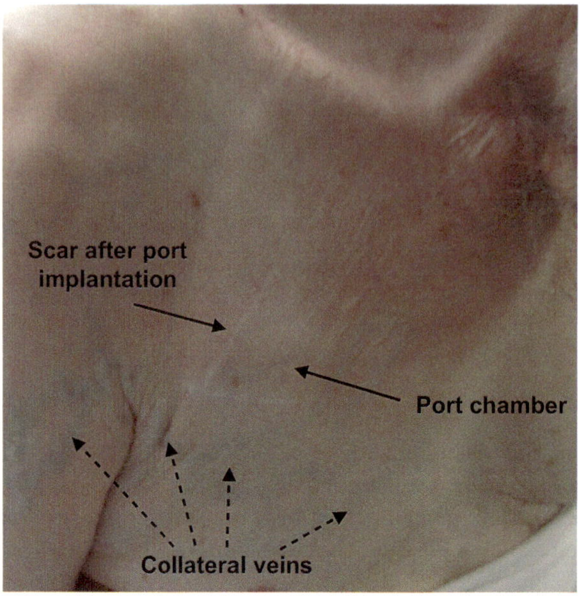

Fig. 13.1 Clinical finding with visible collateral veins in thrombosis of the subclavian vein due to an indwelling port catheter system

Diagnostics

- Assess Wells score!
- Clinical examination
  - Examination findings are usually already sufficient
  - Difference in circumference and doughy-edematous swelling
  - Tenderness on pressure along the course of the veins
  - if applicable, also visibly increased venous markings prepectorally
- Sonography
  - Compression sonography is usually sufficient
- Chest X-ray a. p.
  - if a port is in place, to rule out dislocation/misplacement
  - Imaging of the upper thoracic aperture (cervical rib, ossifications)
- CT
  - if the extent toward the center cannot be reliably assessed
  - if there is suspicion of a passage obstruction (TOS or malignancy)
  - if there is suspicion of pulmonary embolism

Therapy

- Conservative
  - Indications:
    possible in most cases with few exceptions

- Procedure:
  Compression
  →Initially wrap the arm (short-stretch bandage)
  →subsequently, medical compression stocking (MCS) class II (23–32 mmHg)
  Note for the prescription: there are two length measurements:
  GC: whole arm = wrist to axilla
  ZG: whole arm with hand
  also available as gloves YB (short fingers) and XB (long fingers)
  Anticoagulation
  →e.g., enoxaparin (Clexane®) 1 mg (=100 IU) per kg body weight twice daily
  →overlapping initiation with phenprocoumon (Marcumar®)
  with normal Quick value, the first three days: 3, 2, 1 tablet, then coagulation check on day 4
  →alternatively, DOACs, e.g., rivaroxaban (Xarelto®)
  15 mg twice daily for 3 weeks, then 20 mg once daily

• Interventional
  - Indications:
    if pulmonary embolism is suspected
    cardiopulmonary instability
    severe pain
    massive swelling
  - Procedure:
    Lysis and, if necessary, percutaneous transluminal angioplasty (PTA)/stent
    →critical indication for lysis due to risk of pulmonary embolism
    →critical indication for stent implantation: risk of stent fracture/dislocation with external compression
    systemic lysis therapy possible in case of pulmonary embolism

• Surgical
  - Indications:
    fulminant pulmonary embolism
    progressive swelling and pain symptoms
    proven passage obstruction
    →cervical rib
    →callus after clavicle fracture
  - Procedure:
    cardiac surgery in case of fulminant pulmonary embolism
    venous thrombectomy
    if necessary, venous reconstruction (bypass, interposition graft)
    resection of cervical rib, clavicle callus, etc.

Call the on-call service at night?

• Usually not necessary, information the following day is sufficient

Tips and Tricks

- Arm vein thromboses are very rare.
- Further outpatient treatment is usually possible.
- The most common differential diagnosis is thrombophlebitis of the superficial arm veins.
- Consider thoracic outlet syndrome (TOS)
- Chest X-ray: cervical rib? Ossifications of the first rib or clavicle?
- If necessary, thrombophilia diagnostics after completion of anticoagulation
- Recommended duration of compression therapy is at least 6 months (prophylaxis for post-thrombotic syndrome)
- Recommended duration of anticoagulation is 3–6 months; with DOACs, overlapping heparin is not necessary, but with Marcumar® it is essential (otherwise risk of paradoxical reaction or "Marcumar necrosis")

Continuation of Case Study

Since the jugular vein on the affected side appears unremarkable, involvement of the superior vena cava is very unlikely. In unclear cases, CT phlebography should be performed. As the patient still needs the catheter, it should be left in place until chemotherapy is completed. Afterwards, prompt follow-up for port explantation should be arranged. Until then, compression therapy and administration of a low-molecular-weight heparin in therapeutic dosage, or, if oncologically appropriate, oral anticoagulation are recommended. The latter can be, for example, rivaroxaban 20 mg once daily.

14 Thrombosis of the Jugular Veins

Jugular vein thrombosis (Fig. 14.1) is most often the subject of consultation requests from other departments (nephrology-dialysis, intensive care unit, oncology); rarely do patients present from outside via the emergency department. Even if there is initially cervical pain, conservative therapy is usually successfully feasible.

Case Example
The on-call nephrologist contacts you from dialysis regarding a female patient who has redness and swelling on her neck, suspected to be due to thrombosis of the internal jugular vein (IJV). He asks, quite agitated, whether a thrombectomy is necessary and requests that you take a look at the patient. On examination, there is redness and swelling on the right side of the neck with moderate tenderness to pressure. You also see the former entry site of the Shaldon catheter, which has since been removed. The right IJV is completely thrombosed, the left is unremarkable and shows respiratory modulation. The patient does not have a fever, and inflammatory markers are within the normal range. What do you do?

Definition
- Thrombosis of the jugular veins
- Usually internal jugular vein (IJV)
- Rarely external jugular vein (EJV)

Typical Patient
- Patient receiving intensive care
- Indwelling or recently removed central venous catheter (CVC) or dialysis catheter (Shaldon)
- Acute or chronic hemodialysis via atrial catheter
- Patient with underlying malignancy (paraneoplastic thrombophilia)

S. Regus, *Vascular Surgical Emergencies*,
https://doi.org/10.1007/978-3-662-72646-4_14

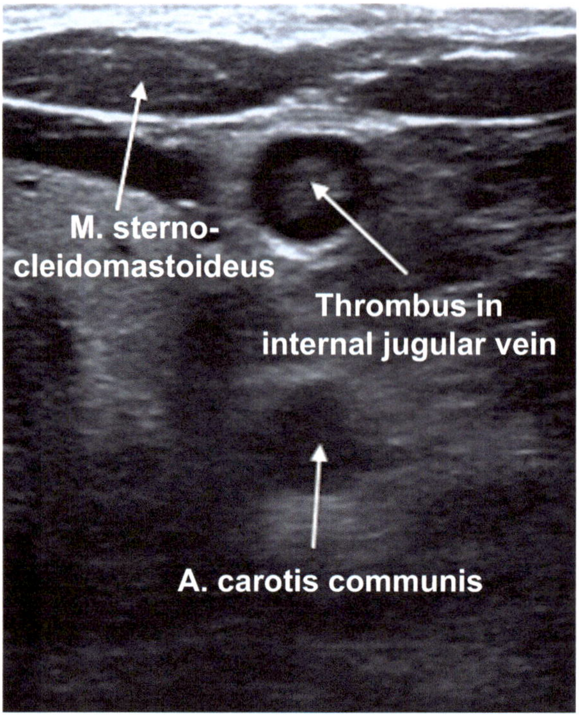

Fig. 14.1 Sonographic depiction of thrombosis of the internal jugular vein

Typical On-Call Situation

- Presentation via emergency department due to neck pain or a painful, reddened cord on the neck
- Consultation from intensive care unit/dialysis
- Patient with dyspnea and suspected or confirmed pulmonary embolism for focus search in the setting of neck swelling
- Dysphagia
- Fever

Diagnostics

- Clinical examination
  - Swelling, redness, induration in the cervical region
- Laboratory
  - D-dimers
  - Inflammatory markers
  - Coagulation parameters
- Ultrasound
  - usually provides sufficient diagnostic information
  - if central outflow cannot be assessed, consider sonographic imaging of the arm veins

  - Respiratory modulation over a compressible subclavian vein virtually excludes a fresh thrombosis of the innominate (= brachiocephalic) vein or the superior vena cava
- CT
  - only in exceptional cases with strong suspicion of central extension
  - workup in suspected pulmonary embolism

Therapy

- Conservative
  - Indications:
    spontaneous thrombosis without foreign body
    regressing swelling and pain
  - Procedure:
    Anticoagulation for 3–6 months
    if necessary, elastic compression bandaging in case of involvement of arm veins or subclavian vein
    cooling in case of thrombophlebitis (ice pack, moist compresses)
    if necessary, antibiotics in case of inflammatory reaction and systemic signs of infection

- Interventional
  - Indications:
    extremely rare
    occasionally appropriate in children in selected cases
    in adults, only in inoperable patients with progressive findings
    Note: high risk of complications
  - Procedure:
    lysis or aspiration thrombectomy
    stent implantation in case of central outflow obstruction (brachiocephalic vein or vena cava)
- Surgical
  - Indications:
    causative foreign body/catheter
    septic dissemination
    increasing compression of the trachea
    severe pain (relative indication)
  - Procedure:
    remove catheter/re-implant on the opposite side
    venous thrombectomy
      → usually unsuccessful
      → high risk of recurrence
    resection of the thrombosed vein
      → in septic thrombosis
      → only in exceptional cases, e.g., septic clinical picture in immunosuppressed patients

Call the on-call service at night?
- Usually not necessary, information the following day is sufficient

Tips and Tricks
- In case of thrombosis of arm veins/axillary/subclavian veins, always assess the internal jugular vein (IJV) sonographically as well
  - If this is also thrombosed, there is a high risk that the thrombosis extends centrally
- If no trigger can be identified, consider malignancy in the differential diagnosis
- An indication for surgery is extremely rare, which often needs to be explained in detail and objectively to colleagues from other disciplines:
  - rarely any benefit for the patient
  - frequent re-occlusion
  - risk of complications
  - good collateralization via other neck veins
- Tumor search (if no other obvious cause)
- Thrombophilia diagnostics after completion of anticoagulation therapy

Continuation of Case Example
You can reassure the patient and your colleague and explain that a thrombectomy is currently not necessary. This would only be required in the event of septic dissemination or involvement of the superior vena cava. Since the IJV on the opposite side is patent, there is no evidence of thrombosis of the superior vena cava. You also do not recommend antibiotics, but instead suggest local cooling and, if necessary, analgesic ointments. In addition, you recommend oral anticoagulation for 6–12 weeks. From your perspective, there is no reason against implantation of an atrial catheter on the opposite side.

Phlegmasia Coerulea Dolens 15

Phlegmasia coerulea dolens (Fig. 15.1) is the only and very serious venous emergency with an indication for invasive therapy. However, differential diagnoses should be excluded and the arterial perfusion status should be carefully evaluated.

Case Example

An 82-year-old female patient is in the emergency department, is being treated by internal medicine, and you are called in for consultation. The responsible internist suspects phlegmasia coerulea dolens, as the patient has a massively swollen and bluish discolored leg. You examine the patient: the left leg is, in comparison to the other side, massively swollen and bluish-livid in color, but warm with prompt capillary refill (<2 s) and palpable foot pulses. On ultrasound, you see a four-level venous thrombosis with the proximal end of the thrombus in the external iliac vein and a respiration-modulated flow signal on the contralateral side. The daughter, who has now arrived, tells you that her mother has an advanced gastric tumor and has refused chemotherapy. What do you write in the consultation note and what do you recommend to your colleague?

Definition

- Extremely rare venous emergency in which massive venous outflow obstruction leads to an increase in compartment pressure above the arterial perfusion pressure
- This results in arterial ischemia, which, like an arterial occlusion of other origin, must be considered an emergency and treated accordingly.

Typical Patient

- Often younger women with thrombophilia
- Left >> right due to the crossing of the left iliac vein under the right iliac artery (May-Thurner!)

S. Regus, *Vascular Surgical Emergencies*,
https://doi.org/10.1007/978-3-662-72646-4_15

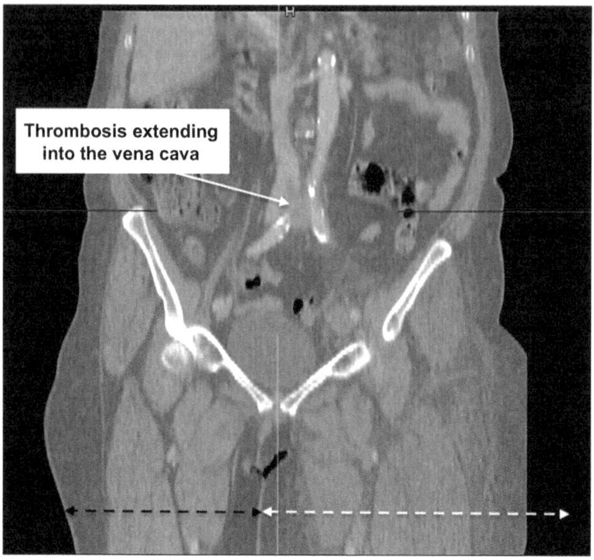

Fig. 15.1 CT with contrast agent (arterial and venous phase) of a female patient with phlegmasia coerulea dolens due to a thrombosis extending into the inferior vena cava. Noteworthy is also the massive swelling and increased circumference of the left leg (white dashed double arrow) compared to the right leg (black dashed).

- Usually additional risk factors (oral contraception, nicotine) or
- Risk situation as a trigger (long flight/car journey, surgery, immobilization)
- Prolonged gynecological surgery in lithotomy position is also considered a risk situation
- Malignant underlying disease (often hematological, sometimes not yet diagnosed)

Typical On-Call Situation
- Presentation to the emergency department with massive leg swelling and bluish discoloration
- Often also from the delivery room, from other wards as a consult, or from oncology
- Patient complains of severe leg pain and swelling as well as a feeling of cold and sensory disturbances

Diagnostics
- Clinical examination
  - pay attention to side differences during examination
    often massive difference in circumference of the affected leg
    pronounced feeling of tension
    tenderness along the course of the deep veins and compartments

sensomotor deficit
temperature difference
- Inspection:
  bluish discoloration
  edematous swelling
- Palpate foot pulses:
  if present, this argues against phlegmasia coerulea dolens
  absent foot pulses are not definitive proof either
- Sonography
  - arterial and venous
- CT angiography/phlebography
  - extent of the thrombosis
  - central extension
  - outflow stenoses (especially iliac and caval)
  - arterial perfusion disorder

Therapy
- Conservative
  - Indications:
    only justifiable if arterial perfusion disorder is compensated and regressing (in this case, however, it is not a phlegmasia coerulea dolens)
  - Procedure:
    elevate limb, elastic compression bandaging
    unfractionated heparin via perfusor or
    LMWH in therapeutic dosage
    after acute symptoms subside:
    → Anticoagulation with phenprocoumon or
    → DOAC
    → compression therapy for at least 1–2 years to prevent post-thrombotic syndrome (PTS)
- Interventional
  - Indications:
    confirmed diagnosis
    timely intervention possible if there is no hyperacute ischemia
  - Procedure:
    thrombolysis
    percutaneous transluminal angioplasty (PTA)/stent implantation
- Surgical
  - Indications:
    confirmed diagnosis and critical ischemia that does not allow any delay
    manifest compartment syndrome
  - Procedure:
    Thrombectomy
    → via the groin
    → thrombectomy of the pelvic veins with Fogarty catheter

→ peripheral thrombectomy mechanically by manual compression and "milking"

if necessary, fasciotomy

→ often not necessary, as swelling usually subsides quickly once thrombectomy is performed

→ if in doubt, however, it is better to have a low threshold for indication and not be influenced by cosmetic considerations

Call the on-call service at night?

- Call, as this is an absolute emergency

Tips and Tricks

- In phlegmasia coerulea dolens, foot pulses are absent!
- A severely swollen and lividly discolored leg is often an impressive and alarming finding, and the suspected diagnosis of "phlegmasia coerulea dolens" is often made out of fear. However, a warm foot with palpable foot pulses rules out this diagnosis and should be a reason for (at least temporary) reassurance
- A "normal" thrombosis practically never leads to phlegmasia. Additional factors almost always have to be present, such as homozygous thrombophilia or a hematological or oncological underlying disease (even if not yet diagnosed)
- Rare, but very serious emergency
- Limb is at risk in the event of delayed therapy

Case Study Continuation

Based on the findings available to you, this is a four-level venous thrombosis in a patient with a malignant and palliatively treated underlying disease. You suspect tumor-induced thrombophilia, but currently see no evidence of phlegmasia coerulea dolens. You recommend, as tolerated by the patient, elastic compression bandaging and anticoagulation with heparin. You are able to reassure both your colleagues and the patient and her relatives, as no surgical intervention is currently necessary. In the majority of cases, the swelling subsides quickly with the above-mentioned measures.

(Ascending) Thrombophlebitis of the Great Saphenous Vein

16

In ascending (ascendant) thrombophlebitis of the great saphenous vein (see Fig. 16.1), the saphenofemoral junction is often not crossed, and conservative therapy is possible. If the junction is involved or crossed, close sonographic monitoring or surgical intervention is necessary to prevent the serious complication of pulmonary embolism.

Case Example

A 54-year-old male patient presents to the emergency department reporting increasing swelling and pain in his left thigh. He has also palpated a thickened cord in the groin and suspected an inguinal hernia. The colleague from general surgery found no evidence of a hernia on ultrasound, but did observe an abnormal structure in the femoral vein and suspected a thrombosis.

Clinically, you see a reddened cord on the left thigh, which is very painful for the patient on palpation. Sonographically, there is a thrombosis of the great saphenous vein over a length of approximately 8 cm, with proximal extension into the common femoral vein (CFV). Here, you see a well-surrounded thrombus cap. The external iliac vein (EIV) is free of thrombus and shows respiratory modulation. The patient has no shortness of breath or other abnormalities. What do you do?

Definition

- Ascending thrombosis of the great saphenous vein, sometimes also the small saphenous vein
- If varicosis is also present, the precise term is varicophlebitis.
- The extent and possible involvement of the deep veins at the saphenofemoral junction are decisive.

Typical Patient

- Usually younger patients, women > men
- Patients often report known varicose veins and previous surgeries

S. Regus, *Vascular Surgical Emergencies*,
https://doi.org/10.1007/978-3-662-72646-4_16

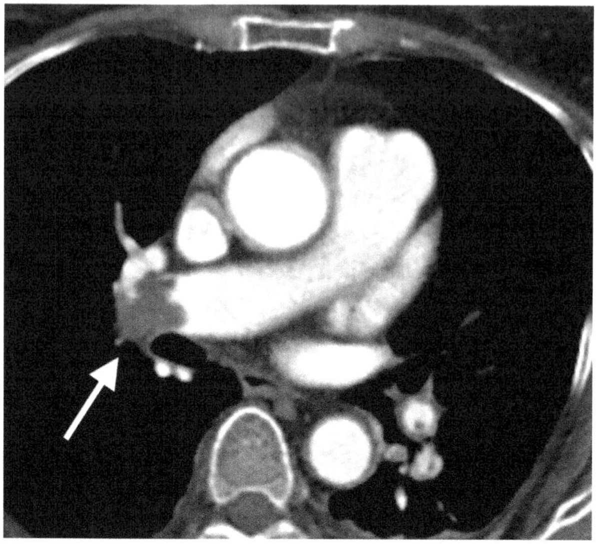

Fig. 16.1 CT with arterial and venous phase shows a fulminant pulmonary embolism on the right (arrow) in a 42-year-old female patient with thrombophlebitis of the great saphenous vein (GSV) extending beyond the saphenofemoral junction

- Presentation due to painful leg swelling
- Fever and wounds are rare

Typical On-Call Situation
- Usually via the emergency department
- Frequently referred by general practitioners with the suspected diagnosis of "thrombosis"
- Sometimes re-presentation after recent endovenous therapy

Diagnostics
- Clinical examination
  - Redness along the course of the vein with
  - localized tenderness
  - painful cord palpable and visible

- Laboratory tests (coagulation, D-dimers, blood count)
- Ultrasound
  - Thrombosis and thickening of the vein wall visible
  - additional edematous soft tissue swelling
  - proximal extension and distance to the saphenofemoral junction or
  - involvement of the junction or deep vein
- ECG
  - if pulmonary embolism is suspected (signs of right heart strain)

- CT
  - if pelvic vein/caval thrombosis is suspected
  - if pulmonary embolism is suspected

Therapy

- Conservative
  - Indications:
    if the saphenofemoral junction is not involved
    if the age of the thrombosis is unclear
    in multimorbid patients
    if surgery is refused
  - Procedure:
    if >5 cm distance:
      →Compression therapy
      initially elastic compression bandaging
      then MKS class II, A-G (thigh-high stocking)
      →symptomatic treatment
      →if necessary, heparin/heparinoid in prophylactic dosage
      e.g., 6 weeks Arixta® (fondaparinux) 2.5 mg/d
    if < 3 cm distance:
      →therapeutic dosage
      →3 months Arixta® (fondaparinux) 7.5 mg/d once daily or
      →oral anticoagulation
    if extending to the saphenofemoral junction:
      →close sonographic monitoring (e.g., after 7 days) or
      →indicate surgery
- Surgical
  - Indications:
    if the saphenofemoral junction is involved or if extending into the deep venous system
  - Procedure:
    simple crossectomy, sometimes with partial removal of the great saphenous vein
    subsequent compression therapy for at least 2 weeks and
    for 3 months Arixta® (fondaparinux) 7.5 mg/d once daily or oral anticoagulation

Call the on-call service at night?

- Usually not necessary, information on the following day is sufficient
- Keep the patient fasting for the ward round, so that surgery can be performed if needed

Tips and Tricks

- The indication for surgery is now set increasingly rarely and more strictly; the trend is toward conservative therapy (compression, anticoagulation)

- Inpatient admission is rarely indicated
  - if the thrombosis extends into the deep venous system and surgery is indicated
  - in case of suspected or confirmed pulmonary embolism
- If surgery, then
  - no complete stripping of the vein, as it is often very indurated and inflamed
  - Postoperative anticoagulation is not strictly indicated, but is advisable in case of doubt, as the deep venous system may be involved via perforating veins despite sufficient crossectomy
- If a CT scan is indicated, ask the radiologist to include the thorax. Information is often lost here, and in the end two CTs (first pelvis/leg, then thorax) are performed with double the radiation dose

Continuation of Case Example

You explain to the patient that although this condition can also be treated conservatively with anticoagulation, due to the risk of pulmonary embolism you recommend surgical management by crossectomy. The patient agrees and you organize the operation (it is already 8:30 p.m., and the patient is not fasting) for the following day. Until then, you prescribe administration of a low-molecular-weight heparin in therapeutic dosage.

17 Thrombophlebitis of the Small Saphenous Vein

Thrombophlebitis of the small saphenous vein (Fig. 17.1) is significantly less common than that of the great saphenous vein and is rarely a reason for emergency presentation. More often, it is the reason for an outpatient visit to the vascular surgery clinic and is usually treatable with conservative measures.

Case Example
A 32-year-old obese female patient with a body mass index (BMI) of 42 already has clinically pronounced varicosis in both lower legs as well as a gaiter-shaped venous ulcer on the right. She complains of pain in her right calf, and her general practitioner suspects a thrombosis. On examination, you already see a very prominent varicose cluster in the right calf with significant surrounding redness, soft tissue induration, and skin involvement ante perforationem. The varicose cluster is not compressible on palpation, and sonography reveals varicophlebitis. However, the deep venous system is patent and shows no evidence of thrombosis. The patient has severe pain over the area of varicophlebitis. What do you do?

Definition
- Thrombosis of the small saphenous vein with or without involvement of the deep venous system
- Usually in the presence of varicose veins (then more correctly referred to as varicophlebitis)

Typical Patient
- Patient (most often overweight women) with known varicose veins
- Often recent surgical treatment of varicose veins, usually endoluminal
- sometimes also current or recently diagnosed deep vein thrombosis of the leg
- Cancer patients with paraneoplastic thrombophilia
- Immobility due to illness or as a result of travel

S. Regus, *Vascular Surgical Emergencies*,
https://doi.org/10.1007/978-3-662-72646-4_17

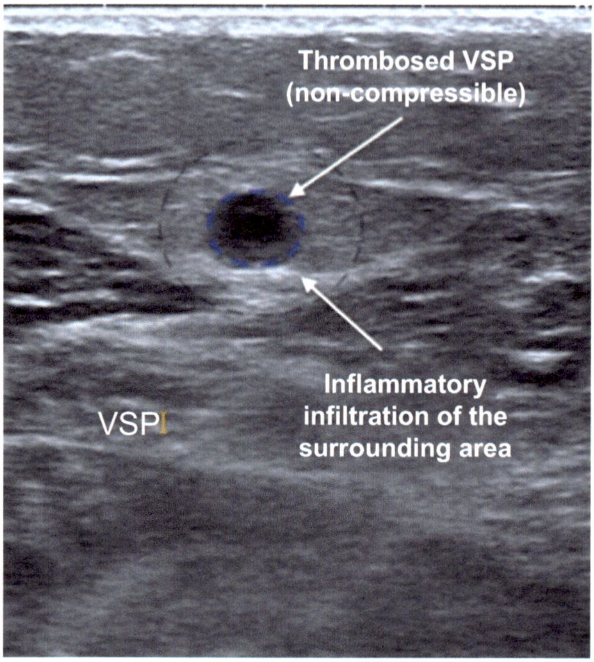

Fig. 17.1 Sonographic image of thrombophlebitis of the small saphenous vein with visible inflammatory infiltration of the surrounding tissue

Typical Situation on Duty

- Often presents to the emergency department due to acute pain
- Rarely as a consult
- Usually outside of on-call hours via the outpatient clinic

Diagnostics

- Clinical examination
  - usually sufficient
  - classic triad of a reddened, thickened, painful cord along the course of the vein
- Laboratory
  - Blood count (leukocytosis? thrombocytosis? anemia?)
  - Coagulation studies
  - D-dimers
- Sonography
  - often already visible in B-mode
  - hypoechoic formation in the distended vein
  - involvement of the deep veins via the saphenopopliteal junction

- Phlebography
  - indicated only in exceptional cases, e.g., after multiple previous surgeries
- CT
  - if the deep venous system is involved, to assess central extension or
  - if pulmonary embolism is suspected
  - not indicated for further evaluation of uncomplicated thrombophlebitis or varicophlebitis

Therapy
- Conservative
  - Indications:
    the vast majority of varicophlebitis and thrombophlebitis cases
  - Procedure:
    Local therapy:
      → analgesic ointments (e.g., Voltaren®)
      → if necessary, heparin-containing ointments (e.g., Thrombophob®)
    Compression therapy
      → by means of elastic compression bandaging or
      → medical compression stocking class II, A-D (knee-high stocking)
      → Duration:
      recommended for at least 2 weeks depending on extent
      in cases of varicosis, possibly long-term
    Anticoagulation
      → not indicated in uncomplicated, distal, short-segment (<5 cm) thrombophlebitis without involvement of the deep venous system
      if necessary, fondaparinux (Arixtra®) prophylactically 2.5 mg once daily
      → in complicated, long-segment, proximal, or deep venous system-involving cases:
      preferably fondaparinux (Arixtra®) 7.5 mg once daily s.c. (therapeutic) or
      e.g., enoxaparin (Clexane®) twice daily, weight-adjusted
      then overlapping with phenprocoumon (Marcumar®)
      alternatively, start directly with a NOAC, e.g., rivaroxaban (Xarelto®) 15 mg twice daily for 3 weeks, then 20 mg once daily
      Duration 6–12 weeks
- Interventional
  - Indications:
    rarely indicated
    primarily elective for treatment of varicosis
  - Procedure:
    endovenous/endoluminal
- Surgical
  - Indications:
    urgent: isolated crossectomy in case of involvement of the deep venous system

elective: recommended in underlying varicosis after resolution of inflammatory symptoms
  - Procedure:
    crossectomy
    if necessary, thrombectomy of the deep vein if the thrombus extends into it
    incision and expression of the thrombus in case of infection and severe pain

Call the on-call service at night?

- Usually not necessary, information the following day is sufficient
- Keep the patient fasting for rounds in order to be able to perform surgery

Tips and Tricks

- Thrombophlebitis of the small saphenous vein is very rare
- Usually occurs after previous varicose vein surgery
- In cases of disseminated involvement (arm, leg, thorax), always consider an underlying malignancy (thrombophlebitis migrans)

Continuation of Case Example

You can either perform local therapy (ointment dressing, mild bandaging, ice cooling) and, if necessary, additional systemic pain management, as well as schedule an outpatient follow-up appointment. Alternatively, you can perform an incision over the thrombophlebitis with expression of the thrombus. However, the latter is sometimes not feasible without pain, as local anesthesia rarely works reliably. This is due to significant soft tissue inflammation. Such a procedure can also be performed under general anesthesia (prone position!), which can be done the following day if the patient is suffering and requests treatment. In principle, the patient can be admitted the next day fasting and fully prepared for surgery. As a precaution (although not evidence-based), administration of a low-molecular-weight heparin in therapeutic dosage is recommended.

Part V
Soft Tissue Infections

18 Foot Abscess in Diabetics

Abscesses in diabetic foot syndrome are a common complication and one of the most frequent reasons why diabetic patients present as emergencies. The general rule, as with all other abscess formations, applies: Ubi pus, ibi evacua (Where there is pus, evacuate it). Due to diabetic polyneuropathy, this can often be performed painlessly in diabetics without anesthesia.

Case Example

What do you do if, in the patient whose foot is shown in Fig. 18.1, the abscess extends from the malum perforans to the middle of the sole and the patient is not fasting?

Definition

- Abscess and infection in "diabetic foot syndrome"
- Deep tissue defects and infections of the foot, primarily caused by diabetic angiopathy and neuropathy

Typical Patient

- Long-standing diabetic with known ulcers and possibly also Charcot foot
- Sometimes younger patients with poor compliance and reduced self-care, as well as poorly controlled diabetes mellitus (high HbA1c, not infrequently even double digits!)
- Fever, chills, poor general condition

Typical Situation on Duty

- Usually presents ambulatory via the emergency department
- Sometimes referred for consultation from other wards (internal medicine!)
- Occasionally presents from dialysis (diabetic nephropathy is the most common cause of dialysis dependency)

S. Regus, *Vascular Surgical Emergencies*,
https://doi.org/10.1007/978-3-662-72646-4_18

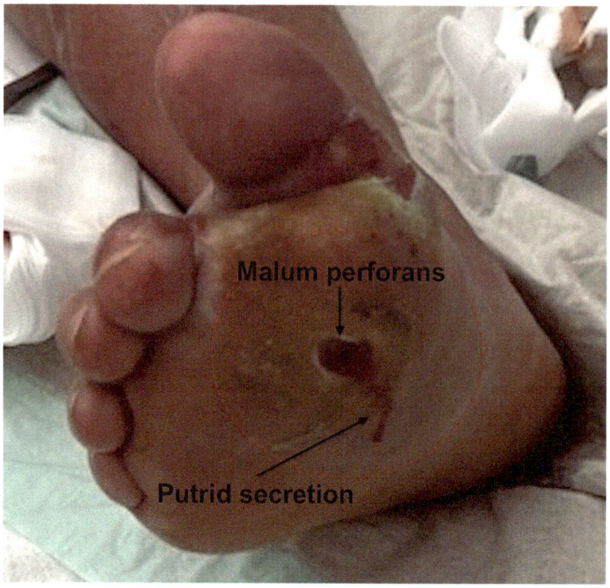

Fig. 18.1 Clinical finding of a plantar abscess in a diabetic patient with malum perforans

Diagnostics

- Clinical examination
  - often diagnosable by smell alone
  - gangrene of one or more toes
  - deep ulcers, extending to bone and joints
  - on pressure, putrid secretion often discharges
  - foot pulses typically strongly palpable (microangiopathy!)
  - sensation often severely reduced (polyneuropathy!)
- Laboratory
  - blood count
  - CRP
  - coagulation
  - renal function and electrolytes
- Swab collection
  - mandatory for: anaerobic and aerobic pathogens
- Determination of ankle-brachial Doppler index (ABI)
  - usually values > 1 (mediasclerosis)
- Ultrasound
  - fluid collection in soft tissues (anechoic)
  - arterial and venous duplex sonography
- X-ray skeleton
  - osteolysis or fractures
  - arthropathy suggests Charcot foot

- CT
  - useful for more precise assessment of bony structures
  - arterial and venous perfusion can also be assessed

- possibly MRI
  - for assessment of soft tissues
  - if the extent is unclear
  - e.g., in suspected ankle joint empyema

Therapy
- Conservative
  - Indications:
    rarely justifiable
    in part, in cases of already spontaneously perforated abscess
  - Procedure:
    Start broad-spectrum antibiotic therapy
      → e.g., piperacillin/tazobactam
      → de-escalation after pathogen identification and receipt of the antibiogram
    antiseptic dressings
    immobilization and rest
- Interventional
  - Indications:
    no meaningful indication regarding the soft tissue findings
    possibly angiography on standby to improve arterial perfusion in cases of crural stenoses or occlusive processes
  - Procedure:
    - percutaneous transluminal angioplasty (PTA) antegrade, possibly even as far as the pedal arteries
- Surgical
  - Indications:
    almost always indicated
    every abscess must be incised (ubi pus, ibi evacua)
    advanced osteolysis
    non-salvageable limb
  - Procedure:
    Abscess drainage and debridement
      → often possible without anesthesia, as there is little pain sensation in diabetic neuropathy
      → all gangrenous tissue should be removed
      sequestrectomy for osteolytically destroyed fragments
      amputation, depending on the extent of the findings
      → border zone
      → toe

→ forefoot
→ midfoot/hindfoot amputation
→ major ablation (lower leg/thigh amputation, knee disarticulation)

surgical vascular reconstruction in proven stenoses/occlusions and after unsuccessful recanalization attempt

→ if the limb is salvageable and
→ exclusion of a septic clinical picture
→ if necessary, in principle up to pedal bypass

Call the on-call service at night?

- Usually not necessary, information the following day is sufficient
- Keep the patient fasting for rounds, so that surgery can be performed if needed
- In cases of severe septic clinical presentation, it is better to call and discuss the procedure

Tips and Tricks

- In the presence of polyneuropathy, abscess drainage up to border zone amputation in the forefoot can often be performed without anesthesia
- Frequent blood glucose monitoring is urgently indicated, as levels are destabilized due to infection
- Internal medicine co-management/interdisciplinary treatment is essential, especially since HbA1c is routinely elevated and patients are multimorbid

Continuation of Case Example

Ideally, you drain the abscess directly in the emergency department without anesthesia and pack the abscess cavity after thorough irrigation. In the majority of diabetic patients, it is possible to drain foot abscesses without any anesthesia. The reason for this lack or absence of pain is diabetic polyneuropathy. In a diabetic foot with abscess, it is therefore quite justifiable to drain it without any anesthesia and, if necessary, perform further procedures (such as toe amputation or sequestrectomy) in the following days. Nevertheless, it is always surprising how much can be done in diabetic patients without any anesthesia.

Phlegmon of the Lower Leg

19

Soft tissue infections such as erysipelas or phlegmon of the lower extremity are also frequently encountered during on-call duty, with conservative therapy usually being sufficient. It is crucial to rule out abscesses and to carefully examine the extremity for the likely entry site of the pathogens.

Case Example
For the patient shown in Fig. 19.1, would you initiate further diagnostic workup (CT or MRI) to confirm or rule out an abscess?

Definition
- Diffuse inflammation of the skin and subcutaneous tissue with local as well as systemic signs of infection
- Bacterial infection, usually gram-positive (streptococci, staphylococci), less commonly gram-negative (enterobacteria) pathogens

Typical Patient
- Often in poor general condition
- Diabetics are more frequently affected, due to immunodeficiency and accompanying microangiopathy.
- Patients with peripheral arterial occlusive disease (PAOD) also have an increased risk, particularly distally and in the foot.
- Obese patients with reduced self-care
- Accompanying thromboses, lipedema and/or lymphedema

Typical On-Call Situation
- Often presents via the emergency department with fever, redness, swelling, and reduced general condition
- Known varicose veins with recurrent inflammation

S. Regus, *Vascular Surgical Emergencies*,
https://doi.org/10.1007/978-3-662-72646-4_19

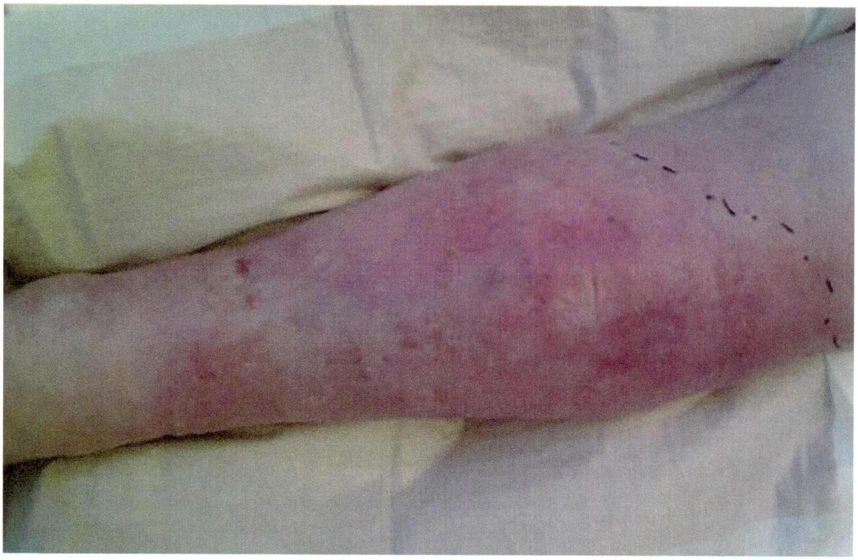

Fig. 19.1 Clinical finding of a phlegmon on the lower leg

- Known wounds and wound infections in risk groups (obesity, diabetes, PAOD)
- Patients after recent varicose vein treatment (in hospital or by a private practitioner)
- Consultation from internal medicine for patients with heart failure and stasis dermatitis

Diagnostics
- Laboratory
  - Inflammatory markers, electrolytes, protein
- Swab
  - in case of open skin injury
  - purulent secretion
- Clinical examination
  - Pulse status
  - Fluctuation/induration
  - Lymphangitis
  - thickened and painful cord (thrombo-/varicophlebitis)
  - edematous swelling
- Ultrasound
  - purulent collection
  - arterial stenoses
  - venous thromboses

- Possibly X-ray in 2 planes
  - in case of localized pressure pain
  - to rule out a recent bony injury
- If necessary, CT
  - only in exceptional cases
  - for example, in suspected activated Charcot foot, osteomyelitis, or deep soft tissue infections

Therapy

- Conservative
  - Indications:
    in cases of diffuse inflammatory infiltration
    when purulent collection has been ruled out
  - Approach:
    Pain management
    Antiseptic dressings
    → e.g., with Octenisept® (octenidine dihydrochloride, phenoxyethanol)
    Antibiotic therapy
    → e.g., Tazobac® 4 g/0.5 g 1–1–1(-1) and/or → clindamycin 600 mg 1–1–1(-1)

- Surgical
  - Indications:
    in cases of purulent collection
    in cases of extensive necrotizing tissue damage
    soft tissue infection involving the fascia
  - Approach:
    Abscess drainage
    Necrosectomy
    Open wound management, if necessary VAC® therapy and subsequent plastic coverage
    Minor amputation
    in extreme cases, major amputation (life before limb)

Call the senior on-call at night?

- As a rule, no
- In cases of pronounced findings, depending on your level of training, independently indicate and perform abscess drainage and necrosectomy
- In cases of sepsis and suspected surgical indication, or if uncertain about the procedure, it is better to discuss by phone and seek confirmation

Tips and Tricks

- Erysipelas and cellulitis are soft tissue infections; in erysipelas, only the skin and very superficial layers are affected, and the visible redness is often striking and sharply demarcated
- In contrast, in cellulitis the visible redness is poorly demarcated and the soft tissue is markedly infiltrated
- The most common pathogens are gram-positive cocci (streptococci, staphylococci)
- Always search for portals of entry

Case Example Continued

These are usually diffuse soft tissue inflammations without a localizable abscess. The latter would also be detectable by sonography. Therefore, performing a CT or MRI scan is not initially indicated. Only in the case of significant clinical deterioration under antibiotic therapy and a localizable fluctuation would there be suspicion of abscess formation and an indication for abscess drainage. However, even in these cases, diagnosis is usually possible by ultrasound.

Acute Charcot Foot

20

The "acute Charcot foot" is a common and serious complication of the diabetic foot syndrome, which may appear clinically rather mild, but in advanced imaging reveals alarmingly profound changes in bone and joint structures.

Case Example
In a 42-year-old patient with type 1 diabetes (Fig. 20.1), both clinical and CT morphology reveal a far-advanced Charcot foot deformity. A malum perforans on the sole of the foot was surgically excised and shows an unremarkable local finding. In addition to intensive diabetological care and blood glucose management, what is, from a surgical perspective, the most important conservative measure to avoid or delay the impending loss of the limb for as long as possible?

Definition
- Acute inflammatory episode of a Charcot foot
- Also referred to as diabetic neuropathic osteoarthropathy (DNOAP)

Typical Patient
- Long-standing diabetic
- Usually still active and in the midst of working life
- No gender preference

Typical On-Call Situation
- Presentation to the emergency department due to
  - swelling of the foot and lower leg
  - subfebrile/febrile temperatures
  - elevated inflammatory markers
- Consultation request from other departments ("Internal Medicine") for focus search in cases of fever/sepsis

S. Regus, *Vascular Surgical Emergencies*,
https://doi.org/10.1007/978-3-662-72646-4_20

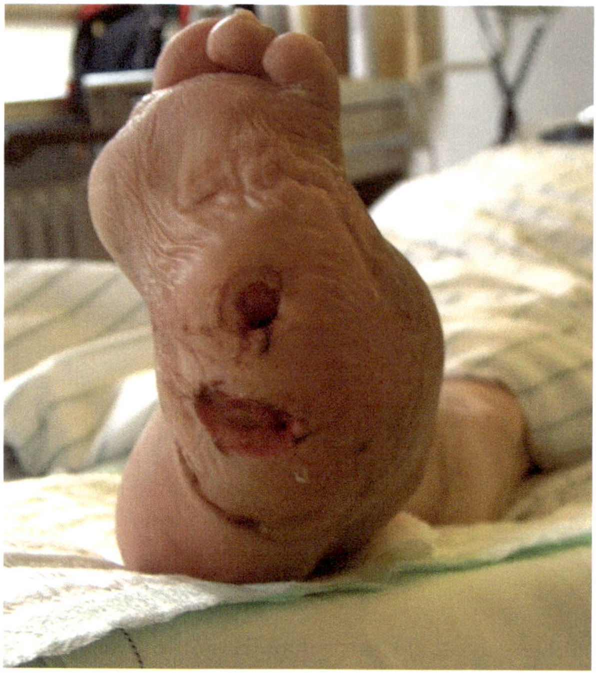

Fig. 20.1 Clinical findings in a diabetic patient with a Charcot foot, showing typical deformities, chronic fistulas, and pressure sores (malum perforans)

  - Here, the foot may appear externally mild and unremarkable.
  - However, one should not underestimate this, as an acute Charcot foot can be hidden behind an externally bland appearance.

Diagnostics

- Laboratory
  - Inflammatory markers
  - Coagulation and platelets
  - Renal retention parameters
- Ultrasound
  - for abscesses in soft tissue
  - or joint empyema
- X-ray
  - Osteolysis
  - Arthrosis
  - Assessment of the joint space
- CT
  - precise assessment of bone structures possible
  - air inclusions as an indication of infection/abscesses

  - arthrosis and both fresh and healing fractures visible
  - with contrast (arterial phase = CTA) for arterial diagnostics
- MRI
  - good for soft tissue assessment
  - visualization of muscles/tendons/ligaments/capsules/cutaneous/subcutaneous tissue
  - less suitable for bone assessment
  - with contrast (= MRA) for further evaluation if peripheral arterial disease is suspected

Therapy
- Conservative
  - Indications:
    often possible
    however, exclusion of an abscess or joint empyema is an essential prerequisite
  - Procedure:
    Antibiotic therapy in case of infection and systemic signs of inflammation
    →Start with broad-spectrum antibiotics, e.g., piperacillin/tazobactam
    →De-escalation once an antibiogram is available

consistent immobilization
    →besides relieving putrid conditions, the most important measure to achieve healing or to prevent progression
    →offloading orthosis is essential
    →often necessary for several weeks, sometimes even months
- Interventional
  - Indications:
    in cases of crural stenoses or occlusive processes
  - Procedure:
    antegrade angiography with readiness for intervention
- Surgical
  - Indications:
    rather rare
    in the presence of an abscess
    advanced osteolysis
    non-salvageable limb
  - Procedure:
    surgical drainage of abscesses
    peripheral bypass reconstruction for long-segment, non-recanalizable stenoses/occlusions
    sequestrectomies
    if necessary, joint arthrodesis (for example, the subtalar joint)
    minor or major amputation if the limb is not salvageable or in case of septic dissemination ("life before limb")

Call the on-call service at night?

- Usually not necessary, information the following day is sufficient
- Keep the patient fasting for rounds to allow for possible surgery

Tips and Tricks

- A combination of diabetic polyneuropathy and microangiopathy can lead to painless (or pain-free) but extremely extensive lesions
- External findings are often bland, while radiologically there may be a surprising (alarming) presentation with extensive osseous destruction
- Arterial reconstructions are rarely indicated, as pedal pulses are usually palpable
- Permanent limb salvage is often not possible and also of little benefit, as the limb becomes increasingly nonfunctional and represents a source of infection
- Consistent offloading is extremely important for limb salvage in acute Charcot foot and should be recommended and implemented long-term (often for several months).
- Even in young patients, amputation should be indicated in a timely manner in cases of sepsis and critical local findings to prevent secondary damage: Life before limb!

Case Study Continuation

Certainly the most important measure to protect and preserve the limb is consistent offloading of the foot. For this, an offloading orthosis is absolutely necessary, as it enables consistent relief of the foot. After the ulceration has healed, custom-made orthopedic shoes are indicated and should be fitted as soon as possible.

Sepsis in Toe Gangrene

21

The complication of sepsis in toe gangrene (Fig. 21.1) is encountered very frequently while on duty and often necessitates urgent toe amputation. Especially in the presence of systemic signs of infection, one should not wait until the next day; even if a vascular imaging and reconstruction is planned, the infected toe should be urgently removed beforehand as the focus of infection and source of sepsis.

Case Example
A 97-year-old female patient from a nursing home is admitted due to a "black toe" on the right. Because of senile dementia, she is not able to provide a medical history. You observe a wet gangrene of the third toe with pronounced surrounding redness; pedal pulses are not palpable on either side, and sonography reveals long-segment occlusions of the superficial femoral artery bilaterally. The patient is bedridden and has flexion contractures in both hip and knee joints. Laboratory tests show elevated inflammatory markers, with a leukocyte count of 18,000/µl. She has a fever with temperatures above 39 °C. What do you do, and what do you recommend to her concerned daughter, who also holds the legal power of attorney?

Definition
- Systemic dissemination of bacterial pathogens in the setting of a foot infection
- Typical pathogens are gram-positive cocci (staphylococci/streptococci) and gram-negative rods (enterobacteria such as E. coli) or pseudomonads (Pseudomonas aeruginosa)

Typical Patient
- Older patient with peripheral arterial occlusive disease (PAOD) stage IV
- Diabetic patients (here, even younger patients may be affected)
- Patients are often severely ill and in poor general condition, as ulcers have usually been present for a long time and the doctor's visit was postponed until the last moment

S. Regus, *Vascular Surgical Emergencies*,
https://doi.org/10.1007/978-3-662-72646-4_21

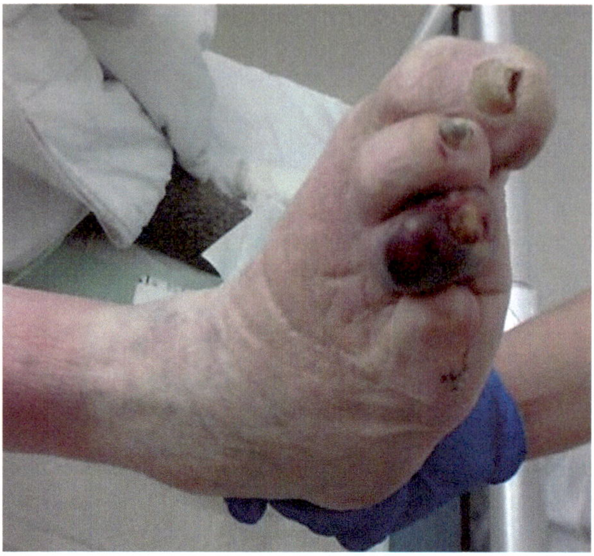

Fig. 21.1 Photo of a wet gangrene of the third toe with phlegmon in a diabetic patient

Typical Situation on Duty

- Usually presents via the emergency department with fever and "black toes"
- Sometimes also as a consult from other departments (especially diabetology!)
- Or as a consult from the intensive care unit in cases of poor general condition and circulatory collapse in a septic clinical picture

Diagnostics

- Laboratory
  - Inflammatory markers such as leukocytes, CRP
- X-ray
  - Are osteolyses visible?
  - Recent or older bony injuries?
- Ultrasound
  - to assess arterial perfusion and
  - the soft tissues (putrid changes)
- MRI/CT
  - only in exceptional cases, for example in suspected ankle joint empyema, Charcot foot, abscess formation

Therapy

- Conservative
  - Indications:
    in cases of dry, superficial gangrene
    usually not sufficient on its own and only as an adjunct to invasive measures
  - Approach:
    Antibiotic therapy
    → initially broad-spectrum
    e.g., piperacillin/tazobactam 4.5 g 1–1–1–1 i.v.
    amoxicillin/clavulanic acid 875/125 1–1–1 orally
    in case of allergy, meropenem 4 × 1 g or clindamycin 3 × 600 mg
    → then de-escalation after receiving the antibiogram
    antiseptic dressings
    immobilization and rest
- Interventional
  - Indications:
    in PAOD to improve perfusion
  - Approach:
    antegrade angiography with readiness for intervention
- Surgical
  - Indications:
    in any deep gangrene
    abscess formation
    in cases of osteolysis
    septic dissemination
  - Approach:
    abscess drainage
    toe amputation
    if necessary, abscess drainage of the sole!
    if necessary, major amputation in extensive findings ("life before limb")

Call the on-call consultant at night?

- Usually not necessary, information the next day is sufficient
- Keep the patient fasting for rounds, so that surgery can be performed if needed

Tips and Tricks

- Antibiotic therapy does not replace abscess drainage, following the principle: "Ubi pus, ibi evacua" ("Where there is pus, evacuate it")
- If the clinical findings are stable, perform vascular diagnostics first
- In cases of wet toe gangrene and septic dissemination, perform amputation first to control the infection, and subsequently, if necessary, improve arterial perfusion (interventionally or surgically)
- In cases of extensive findings and a non-salvageable limb: indicate major amputation, otherwise there is a risk to the patient's life

Continuation of Case Example

In view of the advanced age, you would refrain from further diagnostics, as they would have no consequence. The theoretically possible creation of a femoropopliteal bypass should be discouraged due to the considerable risk of complications and the questionable benefit for the patient. You recommend amputation of the inflamed toe and explain to the daughter that, due to the deteriorated blood supply, the wound may not heal. In that case, a thigh amputation might also become necessary in the course of treatment, but you currently wish to spare the patient from this.

Part VI
Atrial and Port Catheters

22 Dysfunction of a Port Catheter

Dysfunction of a port catheter is one of the most common consultation requests from the "chemo outpatient clinic," where often a new puncture and needle replacement are sufficient. If all conservative measures are unsuccessful, surgical revision becomes necessary; however, a chest X-ray should be performed beforehand to assess the catheter position.

Case Example

You are consulted for a female patient whose port is no longer functioning. You examine the patient; the port appears completely unremarkable externally, and the needle seems to be correctly positioned. Nevertheless, you decide to reposition it, which is accomplished without difficulty. However, the port remains neither flushable nor aspiratable. It was implanted two years ago. You order a chest X-ray, which shows that the tip of the port has flipped upward into the jugular vein. In a previous image from a year ago, the tip was correctly positioned. The catheter is still needed for chemotherapy and therefore cannot simply be removed without replacement. What do you do next?

Definition

- Non-functioning port catheter
  - either due to dislocation of the chamber (Fig. 22.1) or the catheter tube or
  - due to thrombosis in the catheter tube and/or the central veins

Typical Patient

- Presentation from the "chemo outpatient clinic" or as a consult from other wards because the port can no longer be punctured or flushed
- Often, the catheter was placed a long time ago (sometimes years)

S. Regus, *Vascular Surgical Emergencies*,
https://doi.org/10.1007/978-3-662-72646-4_22

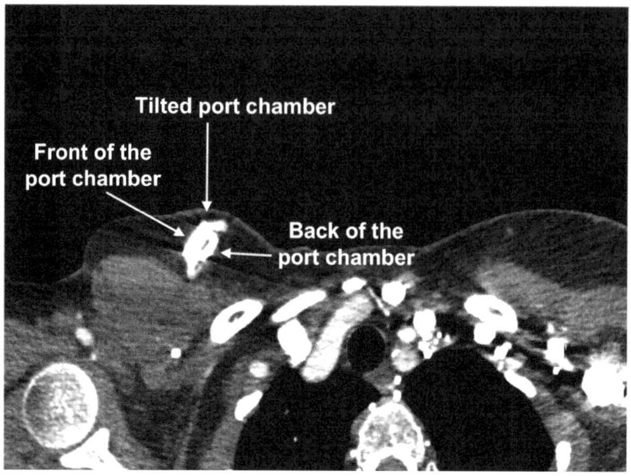

Fig. 22.1 CT shows a tilted port chamber as the cause of port dysfunction with unsuccessful puncture attempts

- But sometimes, implantation was only recently performed, with suture material still in situ
- Occasionally, signs of infection with fever and chills

Typical On-Call Situation
- Chemotherapy, infusions, or nutrition are not possible
- Huber needle (the right-angled special needle) is often in place
- Possibly visible external redness
- Sometimes also extravasation after failed puncture and infusion into the subcutaneous tissue

Diagnostics
- Clinical examination and functional testing
  - Inspection of wound and scar conditions
  - If a Huber needle is in place, check whether it is correctly positioned; if necessary, reinsert.
  - Check whether the catheter can be flushed. Aspiration often does not work, even if the catheter is correctly positioned. Flushing (sometimes initially with gentle pressure) is often successful, and infusion can then be administered without problems.
  - If the needle is correctly positioned and flushing is not possible, dysfunction is present and further measures/investigations are necessary.

  Often, there is significant resistance when attempting to flush the catheter, until the syringe comes loose and the flush solution is expelled—to the dismay of those standing nearby.

- Laboratory
  - Inflammatory markers
- Ultrasound
  - if infection/retention is suspected
  - often clearly visible echo-free formation in the port pocket
  - if necessary, under ultrasound guidance, puncture or spread and obtain secretion for swab
  - however: do not indiscriminately spread the wound or puncture the pocket, as this can lead to contamination
- Chest X-ray a.p.
  - Here you can see the port chamber, the tube, and the position of the catheter tip.
  - If the catheter tip is flipped upward (into the ipsilateral jugular vein) or to the opposite side (contralateral subclavian vein), it is important to know how long the catheter has been in place.

    If only recently, it is usually a technical error during implantation, and surgical revision is possible without further diagnostics.

    If the catheter has been in place for a long time and has always functioned without problems, it is often the case that the catheter tip has become dislocated over time due to central thrombosis or stenosis in the area of the subclavian, brachiocephalic, or superior vena cava.

  : In these cases, it is recommended to perform a
- CT angiography or phlebography
  - This shows whether the brachiocephalic vein or superior vena cava is thrombosed.
  - This is important to avoid intraoperative surprises if the catheter can no longer be placed ipsilaterally.
  - If the cause of the malposition is an ipsilateral thrombosis in the area of the central veins, reimplantation is recommended on the opposite side or ipsilaterally (if the brachiocephalic vein is patent) via the jugular vein.

Therapy
- Conservative
  - Indications:
    in case of incorrect needle placement
    when the port is no longer needed
  - Procedure:
    perform a new puncture
    change the needle
    a port that is no longer needed may, in exceptional cases (e.g., coagulation disorder, explicit patient request), be left in place temporarily, but in principle should be removed as soon as possible
- Interventional
  - Indications:
    suspected port thrombosis

  - Procedure:
    Instillation of rtPA (Actilyse®) and heparin mixture
    →1 mg Actilyse®/1000 IU heparin
    →usually 5 mg Actilyse® with 5000 IU heparin
- Surgical
  - Indications:
    definite malposition
    not recanalizable by lysis
    port no longer needed
    suspected infection
  - Procedure:
    explantation
    if necessary, replacement on the same side or
    new placement on the contralateral side
    if infection is suspected, administer antibiotics and, if necessary, temporarily place a central venous catheter (CVC) for bridging

Call the on-call service at night?
- Usually not necessary, information on the following day is sufficient
- Keep the patient fasting for the ward round in order to be able to perform surgery if needed

Tips and Tricks
- Often, correcting the needle is sufficient
- Do not forget chest X-ray before proceeding to surgical revision
- A catheter that has migrated cranially or has flipped upwards into the internal jugular vein may indicate stenosis/occlusion of the superior vena cava
- Do not puncture the pocket or spread the wound indiscriminately (risk of infection!)
- Since port explantation (in contrast to implantation) does not require special facilities, the port can usually (depending on the standards of your own hospital/department) be explanted by the on-duty resident in the procedure rooms of the emergency department

Continuation of Case Example
In principle, you could indicate surgical revision and new placement; in the simplest case, repositioning the tip would be possible. Nevertheless, it is strongly recommended to order a CT scan preoperatively to determine the cause of the dislocation. Often, a thrombosis of the superior vena cava is the underlying issue, which can lead to surprises and complications during surgery. In some cases, a radiological intervention (e.g., stent angioplasty of the superior vena cava) may even be necessary beforehand.

23 Infection of a Port Catheter

Often clear signs of infection and putrid secretion, but sometimes only mild local findings and fever during infusion therapy. In case of doubt, it is better to remove an infected port catheter (Fig. 23.1), which can be done under local anesthesia in treatment rooms of the emergency department or outpatient clinic.

Case Example
A 35-year-old patient with a port for nutrition due to short bowel syndrome is referred to you for consultation with the request to remove the port because of a suspected infection. The port is still needed; if removed, a temporary central venous catheter (CVC) would be required and planning for port placement on the opposite side would be necessary. Externally, the port appears completely unremarkable, but the patient is in a very poor general and nutritional state and tells you that he repeatedly has fever in the evenings. He does not see any connection with the infusion or the nutrition via the port. He has had the port for 2 years and is afraid that it will have to be removed and that he will need another operation. He asks you if there is any alternative to removing the port. What do you answer?

Definition
- All infections associated with a port catheter

Typical Patient
- Recently implanted port catheter with wound healing disorder, sometimes with residual suture material
- Both cachectic and obese patients are at risk.
- A port used for nutritional therapy is significantly more susceptible than one used for chemotherapy, as the "nutrition port" is virtually always accessed and the needle remains in place permanently.

S. Regus, *Vascular Surgical Emergencies*,
https://doi.org/10.1007/978-3-662-72646-4_23

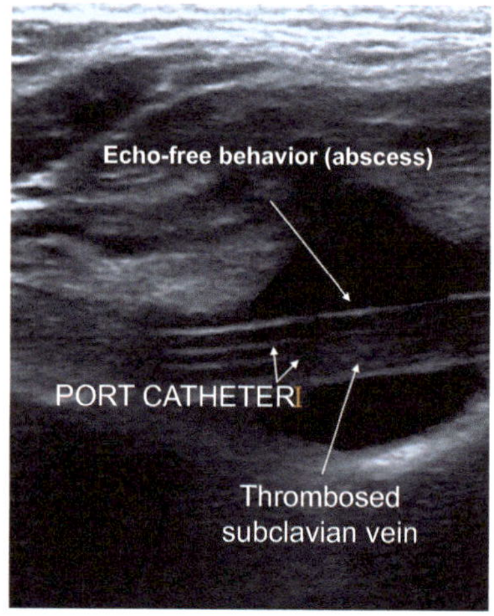

Fig. 23.1 Ultrasound image of an infected port catheter with an anechoic area around the catheter

Typical On-Call Situation

- Patient presents to the emergency department with problems at the surgical wound site after port placement
- "Pus" from the surgical wound (but sometimes only a fibrin-covered wound)
- Consultation request for patients with fever and "positive blood cultures" with an indwelling port catheter for further focus search
- Presentation from "chemo outpatient clinic" with fever during use of the catheter

Diagnostics

- Clinical examination
  - Inspection is often sufficient in clear cases of infection
  - an unremarkable local finding does not rule out infection
- Laboratory
  - Inflammatory markers
  - Blood culture

    if necessary, blood cultures separately from the periphery and the catheter ("Time to Positivity", TTP):

    →especially helpful in cases with mild external findings and positive blood cultures, to prove or rule out a catheter infection

    →Principle: simultaneous collection of blood cultures from the periphery and the catheter and documentation of which sample becomes positive first

    →periphery first: catheter infection unlikely

    →port first: catheter infection likely; even with mild local findings, explantation should be performed
- Chest X-ray
  - Visualization of catheter position, especially the tip
  - important in cases of catheter dysfunction

Therapy

- Conservative
  - Indications:
    mild local findings
    without systemic signs of inflammation and with negative blood cultures
    bridging the time until bacteriological results are available
  - Approach:
    Antibiotic therapy, initially broad-spectrum (e.g., piperacillin/tazobactam 4 g/0.5 g 3 times daily), de-escalate after receiving the antibiogram
    if necessary, "port lock" with antibiotic, taurolidine (Taurolock®), ethanol 70%, or citrate (Citra-Lock®)
    if necessary, local antiseptic dressings
- Surgical
  - Indications:
    in clear cases with
      →pus discharge
      →wound dehiscence
      →pocket infection
    blood culture positive earlier via port than peripherally (keyword: TTP)
  - Approach:
    Port explantation
    Pocket revision
    if a central line is still needed, possibly bridge with a CVC on the opposite side
      →preferably via the internal jugular vein
      New implantation on the opposite side
      →after stabilization of wound conditions and resolution of local and systemic signs of infection
      →via the cephalic or subclavian vein

Call the on-call attending at night?

- Usually not necessary, information the following day is sufficient
- Keep the patient fasting for rounds in order to be able to perform surgery if needed

Tips and Tricks

- Not every so-called "port infection" is truly one and necessitates explantation
- Often, it is a simple wound healing disorder that can be treated conservatively, or a fever of another origin
- However, do not underestimate it, as in immunosuppressed patients a port infection can present atypically and mildly, and delayed explantation can quickly become life-threatening
- Do not aspirate seromas in the surgical area shortly after the procedure, as this can provoke contamination and infection

- In case of doubt, poor general condition, no other source of infection, and unsuccessful conservative therapy, the indication for explantation should be made generously
- Since port explantation (in contrast to implantation) does not require special facilities, the port can usually (depending on the standards of your own clinic/department) be explanted by the on-call resident in the procedure rooms of the emergency department

Case Example Continued

Since the port catheter in this case is externally completely unremarkable and there is no evidence of infection, blood cultures should be taken (ideally if the temperature rises again) from both the port and the periphery. If a pathogen is first detected in the peripherally drawn blood cultures, this suggests another source of infection and argues against a port infection. In such cases, administration of antibiotics and a search for the source of infection would be indicated.

The situation is different in the case of clear clinical signs of a port infection (e.g., redness, swelling, purulent discharge from the port site) or if blood cultures are first positive from the port and then from the periphery. In that case, the patient cannot avoid port explantation, and you would need to explain to him that otherwise he would be at high risk of sepsis with a potentially fatal outcome.

Infection of an Atrial Catheter

24

Infection is a common complication of non-tunneled catheters, less frequently (but still regularly) seen with tunneled catheters with cuff. Local findings are often mild, but in cases of doubt and with a typical history (fever during dialysis!), it is better to explant a catheter once too often and too early (Fig. 24.1) than to endanger the patient with a prolonged infection.

Case Study
A 78-year-old hemodialysis patient has had a fever for several days, notably always during dialysis. The dialysis catheter appears unremarkable externally, but the patient is in a very poor general condition, and the nephrologist requests urgent explantation of the atrial catheter. What do you do?

Definition
- Infection of an atrial catheter
- Either as part of a surgical wound infection, by contamination, or by systemic dissemination

Typical Patient
- Often a long-term indwelling catheter in end-stage renal failure
- Typically, however, also recently implanted with suture material still in place, then usually a perioperative infection
- Shaldon catheters or tunneled "uncuffed" catheters (now rarely available) are more frequently affected than "tunneled" Demers catheters with a "cuff"

Typical On-Call Situation
- Consult from dialysis or other wards (usually "internal medicine") due to suspected Demers infection
- Typically, fever during dialysis or

S. Regus, *Vascular Surgical Emergencies*,
https://doi.org/10.1007/978-3-662-72646-4_24

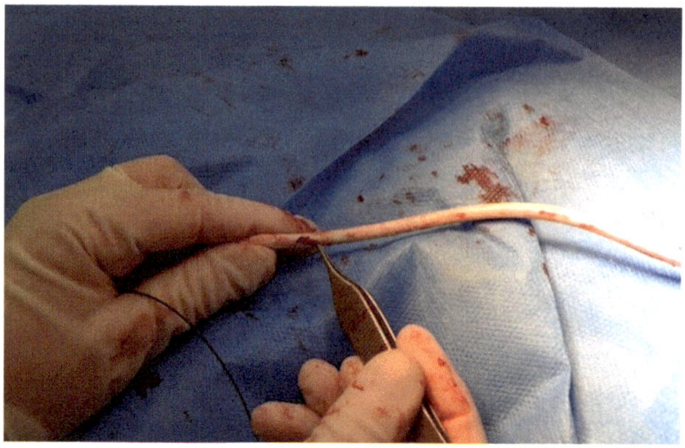

Fig. 24.1 Explantation of an infected Demers catheter with organized thrombus at the catheter tip

- Wound infection with "pus" (note: always examine first, suspected pus is often just a fibrin coating)
- Presentation via emergency department/clinic after Demers implantation and now wound infection and fever

Diagnostics
- Clinical examination
  - Carefully inspect the wound or scar!
  - do not forget: also inspect/palpate the catheter tract (fluctuation? crepitation?)
- Laboratory
  - Inflammatory markers
  - if necessary, blood cultures separately from peripheral vein and catheter ("time to positivity", TTP).
  - particularly helpful in cases with unremarkable local findings and positive blood cultures, to prove or rule out a catheter infection
  - Principle: simultaneous collection of blood cultures from the periphery and the catheter, documenting which sample becomes positive first
    →periphery first: no catheter infection; another source of infection
    →port first: catheter infection likely; even with mild local findings, explantation should be performed
- Swab
  - especially in cases of secondary wound healing and putrid secretion
  - but do not puncture indiscriminately or even spread intact wounds just to obtain material for microbiology
- Ultrasound
  - hypoechoic or anechoic findings along the catheter tract

- Chest X-ray
  - Visualization of catheter position, especially the tip
  - important especially in cases of catheter dysfunction

Therapy

- Conservative
  - Indications:
    with unremarkable external findings and negative blood cultures
    with positive blood cultures, but only or first positive from the periphery
    if fever is completely independent of dialysis
  - Approach:
    Antibiotic therapy, initially broad-spectrum (e.g., piperacillin/tazobactam 4 g/0.5 g 3× daily), de-escalate after receiving the antibiogram
    if necessary, "catheter lock" with antibiotic, taurolidine (Taurolock®), ethanol 70%, or citrate (Citra-Lock®)
- Surgical
  - Indications:
    with clinically clear findings
    with recurrent fever during dialysis and
    with positive blood cultures (TTP: catheter before periphery)
    with questionable infection, if the catheter is no longer needed
  - Approach:
    Catheter explantation
    Leave the wound open
    if necessary, Shaldon catheter on the opposite side and subsequent placement of a new tunneled, cuffed catheter

Call the on-call specialist at night?

- Usually not necessary
- The removal of an infected catheter can usually be performed after a single instruction even without specialist support:
  - The cuff must be dissected free, after which the catheter can usually be removed effortlessly.
  - The "uncuffed" catheter can simply be pulled out.

Tips and Tricks

- "Pus" is often fibrin coating
- Do not explant prematurely if the surgical site appears unremarkable; first rule out other sources of infection
- But do not wait too long either! Dialysis patients are often multimorbid and immunosuppressed
- If there are recurrent fever episodes during dialysis and a marked deterioration in the patient's general condition, prompt explantation should be pursued and a catheter implanted on the contralateral side in the course of treatment

Case Example Continued

When the synthetic material is colonized by bacteria, which may appear externally unremarkable, fever typically occurs during catheter dialysis. In such cases, it is advisable to remove the central venous catheter promptly, without further discussion or time-consuming diagnostics. Dialysis patients are usually multimorbid and can rapidly develop septic complications from infections, which are not infrequently fatal.

Part VII
Dialysis Shunts

25 Shunt Occlusion

Shunt occlusion is a common reason for contacting vascular surgery while on call. If the shunt is not completely occluded, a percutaneous intervention can quickly restore the patient's ability to undergo dialysis under outpatient conditions (Fig. 25.1).

Case Example

It is a typical Friday afternoon, the emergency department is overcrowded, including a 63-year-old dialysis patient whose native Cimino shunt has been occluded since today. He is fasting, his potassium level is slightly elevated, and the nephrology colleague states that hemodialysis is necessary today, or at the latest the following day (Saturday). Would you place a Shaldon catheter in this patient and dialyze him through it in order to perform the surgery on Monday?

Definition

- Occlusion of a hemodialysis shunt
- Usually acute and complete, sometimes incomplete in the case of stenoses

Typical Patient

- Patient undergoing hemodialysis therapy
- Often has been on dialysis via the shunt for many years, but sometimes the shunt was only recently created
- Many patients are well known and regularly present with a shunt occlusion.
- Some patients report that dialysis has not been working properly for several weeks, takes too long (suggesting an arterial inflow problem), or that after needle removal, prolonged compression is required (suggesting a central outflow problem).

S. Regus, *Vascular Surgical Emergencies*,
https://doi.org/10.1007/978-3-662-72646-4_25

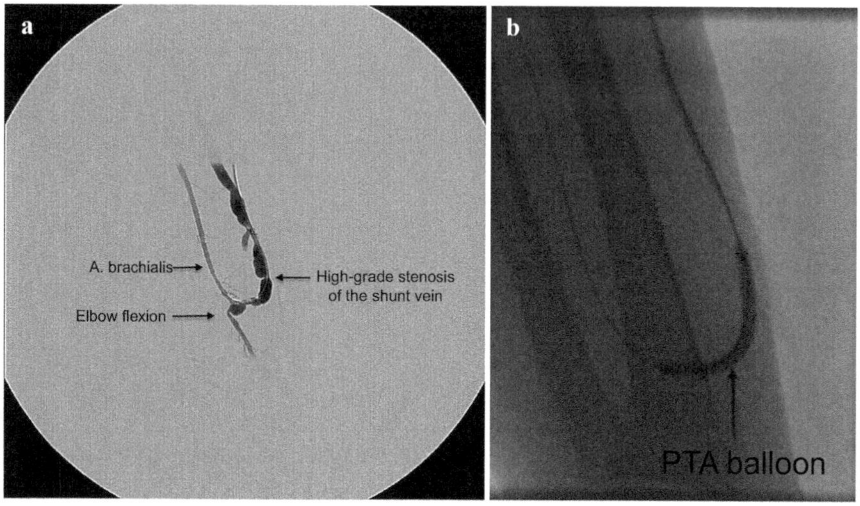

Fig. 25.1 a, b **a** The angiographic image of a patient with a native AV shunt that is no longer suitable for dialysis shows a severe stenosis near the anastomosis as the cause. **b** This was then successfully treated with balloon angioplasty.

Typical On-Call Situation

- Patient with acute shunt occlusion announced from dialysis
- Some patients also notice themselves that the shunt is occluded (no palpable thrill) and present to the emergency department/clinic.
- Sometimes there is also an acute complication such as shunt rupture or bleeding from an aneurysm.

Diagnostics

- Medical history
  - Whenever possible, it is advisable to briefly consult with the "dialysis physician" or nursing staff and inquire about the patient's history.
- Clinical examination
  - Shunt neither has a thrill nor is pulsatile
  - if applicable, a pulse may still be palpable at the anastomosis
  - often palpable indurations along the puncture tract, sometimes aneurysms are visible/palpable
  - usually sufficient to make the diagnosis
- Ultrasound
  - can be attempted to more precisely determine and visualize the cause (stenosis, aneurysm, infection, partial thrombosis, occlusion of the supplying artery)
- Shuntography
  - may be indicated if the anastomosis region is open and there is a downstream partial occlusion or significant stenosis

  - not indicated for diagnostic purposes alone, but only when intervention is planned
- CT phlebography
  - rarely necessary, but useful if central stenosis is suspected
  - important if, in addition to shunt revision, placement of an atrial catheter is planned or necessary. This allows preoperative visualization of central stenoses or occlusions that could complicate atrial catheter implantation.

Therapy

- Conservative
  - Indications:
    possibly in cases where hemodialysis is no longer indicated
      →recovery of renal function
      →functioning transplant kidney
    planned switch to peritoneal dialysis or
    in terminally ill patients
  - Procedure:
    if necessary, CPS powder (1–2 sachets) in case of hyperkalemia
    fluid restriction
    if necessary, loop diuretics if residual function is present
    symptomatic therapy (antiemetics, analgesics, morphine infusion pump) in palliative situations
- Interventional
  - Indications:
    if the shunt is still open at the anastomosis and not completely occluded distally
    if there is a short-segment thrombotic occlusion
    intraoperatively in cases of central stenoses
  - Procedure:
    shuntography and percutaneous transluminal angioplasty (PTA) of stenoses
    treat central stenoses with stent placement if necessary
    lysis therapy with rtPA followed by intervention for unmasked stenoses
- Surgical
  - Indications:
    in cases of complete long-segment occlusion
    in cases of occlusion not amenable to interventional recanalization
    in cases of large aneurysms with a high thrombus burden
  - Procedure:
    if the diagnosis is clear, perform shunt revision promptly, ideally on the day of admission, followed by hemodialysis via the shunt
    if potassium levels are too high and preoperative dialysis is necessary, place a Shaldon catheter and operate the following day
    if the shunt is no longer salvageable (completely exhausted, infection, recurrent occlusions at increasingly shorter intervals), it is advisable to create a

new shunt (preferably autologous and ipsilateral), including implantation of a permanent tunneled atrial catheter (Demers catheter)
alternatively, consider another dialysis modality (peritoneal dialysis)

Call the on-call service at night?

- Depending on the department's standards
- In principle, emergency revision is not indicated, but is performed by some (even at night)

Tips and Tricks

- Aim to perform shunt revision as soon as possible (but not necessarily at night)
- Placement of an atrial catheter should be avoided
- Bleeding and infections are rare, but often complex to manage when they do occur
- Before revision, make a plan as to whether and where the puncture segment can be preserved. Avoid exposing the entire length of the shunt if possible

Case Example Continued

As a general rule, whenever possible, the placement of an atrial catheter should be avoided, as in this specific case. This is associated with an increased risk of infection and not infrequently with thrombosis of the central veins. Therefore, surgical revision should be performed on Friday evening, or at the latest on Saturday morning. In many cases, the anesthesiologist agrees with this approach and the patient is fit for anesthesia if appropriate conservative therapy for potassium control (usually CPS powder) is administered. Under no circumstances should Shaldon catheters be placed indiscriminately in order to schedule the surgical procedure during regular working hours.

Shunt Bleeding

26

One of the most common emergency consult requests from dialysis, in addition to acute shunt occlusion, is shunt bleeding, which is usually due to increased venous pressure. Typically, bleeding complications occur after removal of the dialysis cannula, with notably prolonged compression times.

Case Example
A 54-year-old patient with end-stage renal failure (Fig. 26.1) receives hemodialysis via a native upper arm basilic vein shunt. An aneurysm has been known for a long time; currently, there is a crust from which blood is now spurting. After 30 minutes of compression therapy, the bleeding has stopped, but the shunt is pulsating. Sonographically, there is a high-grade stenosis behind the aneurysm in the mid-upper arm; the basilic vein above this is collapsed but patent. The patient is eager to go home. What do you do?

Definition
- Bleeding or bleeding complication from an arteriovenous dialysis access

Typical Patient
- Patient with a newly created shunt, usually bleeding from the anastomosis area
- Known puncture aneurysm along the shunt
- Progressive ulcer over the shunt
- Multiple shunt interventions in the past due to central outflow problems

Typical On-Call Situation
- Patient referred from dialysis with uncontrollable bleeding after puncture
- Usually already known to have high venous pressure due to central stenosis

S. Regus, *Vascular Surgical Emergencies*,
https://doi.org/10.1007/978-3-662-72646-4_26

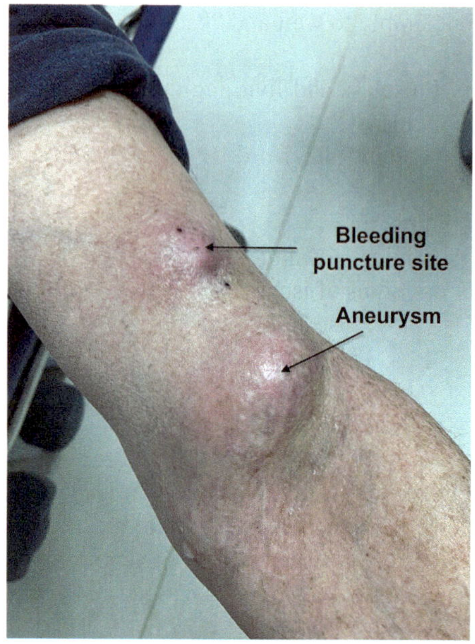

Fig. 26.1 Clinical finding of a recurrently bleeding shunt with aneurysms and central stenoses in the area of the cephalic vein junction (currently no bleeding after adequate compression)

- Patient from angio suite during or shortly after intervention due to rupture as a complication during/after intervention
- Via emergency department with bleeding complication from shunt after recent surgery, known aneurysm with ulceration, or known central outflow problem

Diagnostics

- Clinical examination
  - Inspection
    active or previous sources of bleeding
    ulcer or scab over the shunt
    redness, swelling, and discharge as signs of infection
  - Palpation
  - strongly pulsating shunt vein as an indication of central stenosis and high venous pressure
  - no thrill and no pulsation if the shunt has occluded during compression for bleeding
- Ultrasound
  - thrombus
  - wall thickening
  - outflow and suspicion of central stenoses
- Shuntography
  - If the shunt is patent and there is suspicion of a central outflow problem, shuntography should be performed with readiness for intervention

Therapy

- Conservative
  - Indications:
    if bleeding stops spontaneously and a central outflow problem has been excluded
  - Approach:
    compression or simple dressing is often sufficient
    antibiotics if infection is suspected
- Interventional
  - Indications:
    persistent bleeding
    known or suspected central stenosis
  - Approach:
    shuntography and percutaneous transluminal angioplasty (PTA) of the outflow tract
- Surgical
  - Indications:
    if bleeding occurs shortly after shunt creation and the anastomosis is affected
    large ulcer
    large aneurysm of the shunt vein
    large hematoma requiring decompression
    impending or manifest compartment syndrome
    prosthesis infection
  - Approach:
    oversewing the bleeding source
    revision of the anastomosis, if necessary, new creation
    ulcer resection and reconstruction, possibly including intraoperative dilation of the central outflow tract
    aneurysm plication or resection and interposition
    hematoma decompression
    fasciotomy
    explantation of an infected prosthesis and creation of a new shunt including atrial catheter to temporarily protect the shunt

Call the on-call consultant at night?

- Often can be temporarily stabilized by compression, but if in doubt, it is better to discuss the findings and procedure by phone

Tips and Tricks

- Causes are often high venous pressure (central stenosis) if the puncture site does not stop bleeding
- Infection, ulcer, or aneurysm are other common causes
- Often there is no more bleeding by the time the patient reaches the emergency department because compression was sufficient

- However, do not discharge the patient lightly; the likelihood of recurrent bleeding is very high
- Surgery under bloodless conditions for aneurysm/ulcer over the shunt is often helpful, as there is less bleeding and the procedure can be performed without assistance during on-call duty
- If the shunt continues to pulsate, it is essential to aim for angiographic visualization of the central outflow. Otherwise, a central stenosis and increased venous pressure can lead to persistent bleeding from the puncture sites

Case Example Continued

It is typical for dialysis patients to want to avoid any unnecessary hospital stays, which is understandable to some extent: they are often enough at dialysis and spend a lot of time in the hospital. Nevertheless, in this case, the patient should definitely be asked to sign a statement refusing inpatient treatment, and be strongly advised to stay. Bleeding can recur at any time, and it is obvious that the shunt has a venous outflow problem. Excision of the ulcer, plication of the aneurysm, and autologous patch plasty (using portions of the resected aneurysm wall) of the downstream stenosis should be performed promptly to prevent further bleeding complications.

27 Shunt Infection

In particular, with alloplastic shunts, infections are a frequent and very serious complication in multimorbid and often immunocompromised dialysis patients.

Case Study

An 82-year-old patient with a forearm PTFE loop shunt implanted 2 years ago (Fig. 27.1) presents clinically with severe redness and swelling along the shunt tract. He also has fever and chills. The blood culture results are not yet available, but inflammatory markers are markedly elevated. What would you do?

Definition

- Infectious complication of a hemodialysis shunt
- May be superficial (cutaneous/subcutaneous) or deep, extending to the shunt
- Possible with native (autologous) shunts, but more common with alloplastic accesses

Typical Patient

- Recently created shunt with wound healing disorder at the surgical site
- Obese or cachectic patient
- Multiple revisions in medical history

Typical On-Call Situation

- Presentation to the emergency department with fever
- Partially already externally visible infectious complication with redness, swelling, and putrid discharge from the wound
- Typically also referred for consultation from dialysis/nephrology due to recurrent fever spikes during dialysis
- Sometimes also unclear infection without a definite focus in the presence of a PTFE shunt ("silent infection")

S. Regus, *Vascular Surgical Emergencies*,
https://doi.org/10.1007/978-3-662-72646-4_27

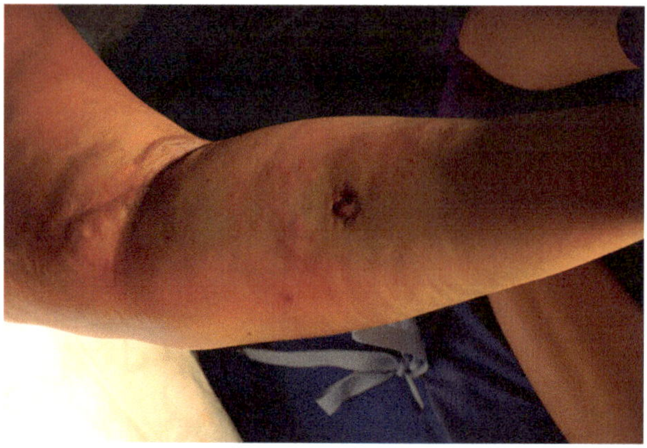

Fig. 27.1 Clinical finding of an infected synthetic shunt with skin perforation and putrid secretion

Diagnostics
- Clinical examination
  - Redness, swelling, induration, putrid secretion
  - Exposed prosthesis
- Laboratory
  - Blood count
  - Inflammatory markers
- Swab
  - in open wounds/secretion
- Blood culture
  - in case of fever/chills
- Ultrasound
  - Hypoechoic collection around the shunt visible
  - Differentiation between collection and aneurysm possible
  - Shunt thrombus/occlusion can be visualized

Therapy
- Conservative
  - Indications:
    rarely promising
    at most for superficial soft tissue infection without prosthesis involvement
    often possible with autologous shunts
  - Procedure:
    Antibiotic therapy (broad-spectrum)
    Local antiseptic therapy (e.g., with Serasept®/Octenisept® or Cutimed sorbact®)

- Interventional
  - Indications:
    no reasonable indication due to infection
    at most in the case of concomitant shunt occlusion and central outflow stenoses
  - Procedure:
    Lysis
    Percutaneous intervention
- Surgical
  - Indications:
    in clear infection with putrid secretion
    in septic clinical picture
    if conservative approach is unsuccessful or
    if signs of infection increase under conservative management
  - Procedure:
    if an attempt to preserve the shunt is justified, a soft tissue revision can be attempted
      →Debridement, abscess drainage, irrigation, VAC application
      →local antiseptic therapy
      →temporary dialysis via central venous catheter and replacement of the infected PTFE segment with autologous or xenogeneic material
    Explantation of the prosthesis and new placement bypassing the infected area
    Shunt placement on the contralateral side
    Abandonment of the access and switch to catheter or peritoneal dialysis

Call the on-call consultant at night?

- Usually, inpatient admission and administration of antibiotics as well as passing on information the following day are sufficient.
- Keep the patient fasting for rounds in order to be able to perform surgery if needed
- In case of bleeding, perforation, or sepsis, telephone contact and discussion are recommended

Tips and Tricks

- The indication for explantation of an infected PTFE shunt should be made liberally
- Conservative therapy is rarely successful
- Patients are at high risk of complications, as they are multimorbid and their immune systems are often weakened
- The dosage of antibiotics ("renal dose") should ideally be discussed with a nephrologist

Case Example Continued

Since the patient clearly has a shunt infection and also shows systemic signs of inflammation, septic dissemination must be assumed and there is an urgent indication for explantation of the shunt. The operation should be performed as soon as possible; the results of the blood cultures do not need to be awaited in this regard.

Part VIII
Vascular Trauma

Traumatic Aortic Rupture

28

Traumatic aortic rupture (Fig. 28.1) is, fortunately, a very rare but life-threatening complication. It is almost always preceded by massive trauma (traffic accident, fall from a great height).

Case Example
A 23-year-old pedestrian is struck by a car and sustains severe thoracic trauma. She is intubated, ventilated, and brought to the trauma bay with moderate hemodynamic stability under the care of an emergency physician. There is suspicion of active bleeding and injury to a major vessel. The mother, who is present at the scene, reports that the patient is pregnant (4th month). The radiologist asks whether CTA diagnostics are still desired. How do you respond?

Definition
- Alternative term: **aortic transection**
- Aortic wall injury due to blunt force with incomplete or complete lesion
- Occurs in the typical location ("aortic isthmus")
- In English-language literature also referred to as "aortic transection"
  - Type I: intimal lesion
  - Type II: intimal and medial lesion
  - Type III: all wall layers, but contained rupture
  - Type IV: open/free rupture

Typical Patient
- Younger patient after traffic accident
  - typically pedestrian or motorcyclist
  - Men >> women
  - Almost always high-velocity trauma (= deceleration trauma, i.e., rapid slowing from high speed)

S. Regus, *Vascular Surgical Emergencies*,
https://doi.org/10.1007/978-3-662-72646-4_28

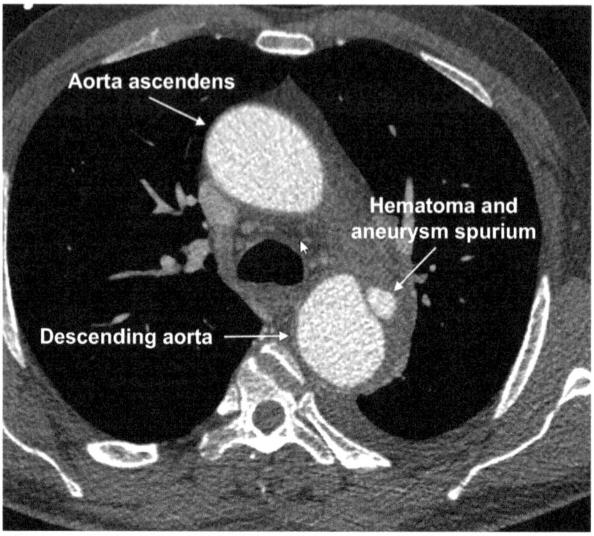

Fig. 28.1 CTA of a type III aortic rupture in a hemodynamically still stable patient shortly before endovascular treatment

- Collision of racing cyclists
- Fall from great height (climbing)
- Skiing accident (downhill)

Typical On-Call Situation
- Announced as polytrauma/thoracic trauma
- With emergency physician via trauma bay
- Often already intubated/ventilated
- Frequently hemodynamically unstable or only slightly stable
- High mortality at the scene (often in type III, almost always in type IV)

Diagnostics
- Clinical examination
  - moderately impaired and few symptoms in type I and some type II lesions
  - severely impaired in type III and in progressive type II lesions
  - Patients with type IV lesions (with rare exceptions) die at the scene
  - Monitor circulatory parameters (pulse, BP, shock index)
  - Assess pulse status
  - Thoracic and sternal hematomas
  - in hemothorax:
    dull percussion note
    auscultatory decreased breath sounds

- Laboratory
  - Blood gas analysis
  - Blood count (anemia)
  - Coagulation
- Ultrasound
  - transthoracic echocardiography
  - if expertise and hemodynamic stability allow, also possible transesophageally and often highly informative
- CT in the trauma bay as a "trauma spiral"
  - often standard as the first diagnostic step in the trauma bay, usually without contrast agent
  - here, one may see irregularity of the aortic wall or a mediastinal hematoma
  - hemothorax
  - possibly retroperitoneal bleeding in the case of additional dissection and extension into the abdomen
- CT angiography
  - with contrast agent ("arterial phase") for more precise diagnostics, often still indicated afterwards
- Diagnostic pleural or peritoneal puncture
  - since widespread use of CT diagnostics, now only indicated in exceptional cases

Therapy

- Conservative
  - Indications:
    with intact vessel wall and no bleeding
    Aortic rupture type I (intimal lesion) and type II (media injury)
  - Procedure:
    intensive care monitoring required
    monitor surveillance
    blood pressure management
    pain management
    laboratory monitoring
    CTA follow-up after no more than 24 h
- Interventional (endovascular)
  - Indications:
    for type II (with increasing size) and
    type III (contained rupture)
    for type IV (open rupture)
    →rarely survived
    →If the patient reaches the hospital in a relatively stable condition, it may be a rupture with extensive adhesions of the soft tissue (e.g., after previous thoracic surgery, chronic inflammatory processes) or a consequence of radiation therapy.

- Procedure:
  endovascular therapy using TEVAR ("thoracic endovascular aortic repair") preferred
  surgical (open)
- Indications:
  Since the introduction of aortic stent grafts, open repair is only performed in absolute exceptional cases (high risk of complications).
  If necessary, as a last resort in unstable patients, also possible in the trauma bay with the primary goal of bleeding control. The patient can then be definitively treated under sterile conditions.
- Procedure:
  sternotomy or thoracotomy
  clamping and suturing
  aortic interposition graft
  mediastinal/thoracic hematoma evacuation
  drain placement

Call the on-call service at night?

- Yes, emergency treatment may be indicated and discussion of findings is absolutely necessary

Tips and Tricks

- Type I can be managed conservatively, type IV rarely reaches the hospital alive
- Even seemingly "harmless" type I lesions must be monitored in intensive care and closely followed up
- In emergency situations, perform CTA even in pregnant women; this is a vital indication as there is a life-threatening risk for both mother and unborn child
- Type II lesions treated conservatively often develop aneurysms over time, so CTA follow-up is necessary
- Do not confuse transection and dissection:
  - Transection (spelled with one "s") means traumatic rupture,
  - Dissection refers to a tear of the intima/media, traumatic or spontaneous.

Continuation of Case Example

Even if pregnancy is present, CT imaging is absolutely necessary for further treatment planning. A confirmed pregnancy is not a contraindication in this case, as there is an acute life-threatening risk for the mother and the unborn child. MRA is not a suitable diagnostic tool in this emergency situation; moreover, its diagnostic value regarding aortic injuries is significantly limited.

Rupture of the Carotid Artery 29

Traumatic rupture of the carotid artery typically results from massive cervical spine trauma, most often in the form of a hyperextension injury. Notably, there is an association with deploying airbags, which can frequently provoke hyperextension.

Case Example
What do you think: Was it necessary to place a shunt intraoperatively in the patient from Fig. 29.1?

Definition
- Tear of the common, internal, or external carotid artery due to blunt or sharp force

Typical Patient
- Usually young men after a traffic accident or high-velocity trauma
- Not infrequently associated with sudden airbag deployment
- Twisting injury/hyperextension
- Occasionally iatrogenic after (unsuccessful) attempt to place a central venous catheter or
- After difficult emergency intubation with hyperextension injury of the cervical spine

Typical On-Call Situation
- Announced by emergency dispatch as polytrauma with vascular involvement, possibly also suspected stroke
- Consultation from the intensive care unit after resuscitation and intubation complication

S. Regus, *Vascular Surgical Emergencies*,
https://doi.org/10.1007/978-3-662-72646-4_29

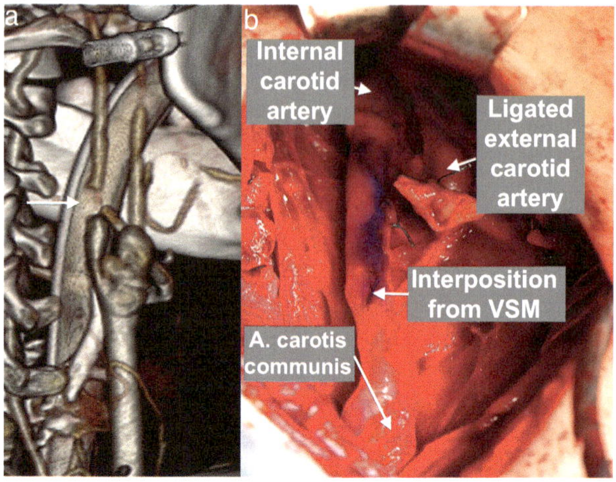

Fig. 29.1 a, b **a** MRA reconstruction of a traumatic avulsion of the internal carotid artery (arrow) in a 28-year-old following airbag trauma. **b** The patient was neurologically unremarkable due to good collateralization via the contralateral side (circle of Willis) and was treated surgically with a venous interposition graft.

- Call from anesthesiologists during induction of anesthesia with suspected arterial malposition of a Shaldon catheter
- Rarely, consultation from neurology due to a stroke and, in further diagnostics, discovery of a pseudoaneurysm

Diagnostics

- Clinical examination
  - large hematoma or pulsatile swelling may already be visible
  - signs of cerebral ischemia possible
  - sometimes a bruit can be auscultated if an AV fistula has formed
  - however, a fistula only develops in a chronic process with subsequent acute rupture
- Ultrasound
  - usually confirms the finding
- CT angiography
  - indicated to confirm the diagnosis

Therapy

- Conservative
  - Indications:
    if no active bleeding is detectable
    with intact vessel wall
    no signs of compression of the airway or esophagus

  - Approach:
    monitoring, on the monitor, possibly also in intensive care
    follow-up diagnostics (CTA) to rule out increase in size
    cooling with ice
    pain management
    if necessary, optimization of coagulation
- Interventional/endovascular
  - Indications:
    contained rupture
    active bleeding
    increase in size
  - Approach:
    covered stent ("covered")
    embolization with coils (practicable only for branches of the external carotid)
- Open surgical
  - Indications:
    in open rupture
    in active bleeding
    compression symptoms (dysphagia, dyspnea)
    malposition of a Shaldon catheter/CVC in the artery
  - Approach:
    oversewing
    hematoma evacuation
    removal of the catheter and suturing of the artery, possibly including patch angioplasty
    placement of an interposition graft (autologous or alloplastic PTFE)

Call the on-call consultant at night?
- Yes, emergency treatment is indicated

Tips and Tricks
- In cases of severe compression symptoms, hematoma evacuation may be necessary before intubation, as the trachea is obstructed and the tube cannot be advanced
- In the case of arterial malposition of a catheter and a contained lesion without bleeding, surgery can, in exceptional cases, be performed the next morning. However, in such cases, therapeutic anticoagulation should always be administered until catheter removal (and possibly beyond), usually with unfractionated heparin

Continuation of Case Study
Due to the obviously very good collateral function, the patient was clinically unremarkable and the placement of a shunt was not necessary. While the first assistant

harvested and prepared the great saphenous vein from the thigh, the surgeon, together with the second assistant, exposed the injured carotid artery and dissected the proximally and distally accessible common and internal carotid arteries. The external carotid artery was ligated to achieve better anatomical conditions. The venous interposition graft could be anastomosed without difficulty, first distally, then proximally, each beveled end-to-end. After confirming good backflow and strong inflow, as well as excluding pre- and post-anastomotic thrombi, the anastomosis was released. Throughout the entire operation, neuromonitoring potentials remained unremarkable, so the placement of a shunt was not necessary. The further postoperative course was uneventful.

Vascular Trauma with Foreign Body In Situ

30

In vascular trauma with a foreign body in situ, this usually involves a foreign object that has been forcibly introduced from outside, either intentionally or unintentionally, most commonly weapons and tools. However, an iatrogenically introduced implant can also lead to a vascular surgical complication (Fig. 30.1).

Case Example
An 83-year-old woman developed a chronic cervical fistula after radiation therapy for laryngeal cancer 2 years ago and a history of stent PTA for a high-grade asymptomatic right ICA stenosis 6 years ago. The stent is visible and, according to the patient's history, has frequently led to bleeding complications. In current imaging, both the stent and the ipsilateral CCA and ICA are occluded over a long segment. The patient shows no neurological deficits, the stent occlusion is longstanding, and occurred asymptomatically. What do you think was the treatment for this patient?

Definition

- Traumatic vascular injury caused by penetrating objects, e.g., arrow, knife, or projectiles
- Erosive bleeding due to iatrogenically introduced implants

Typical Patient

- More common in large cities with hotspots such as drug scenes, etc.; less common in rural areas
- Accidental injury during sports (archery, fencing) possible
- Occupationally exposed individuals can be easily injured, e.g., falling from scaffolding onto sharp objects or axe injuries among forestry workers.
- In leisure time after violent altercations, for example in fights or at large sporting events

S. Regus, *Vascular Surgical Emergencies*,
https://doi.org/10.1007/978-3-662-72646-4_30

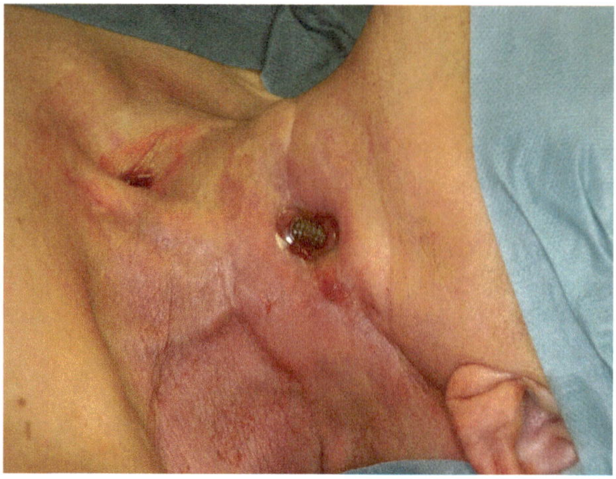

Fig. 30.1 Clinical finding of an exposed stent of the left common carotid artery

- Very often under the influence of alcohol and/or drugs
- Men >> women

Typical Situation on Duty
- Almost exclusively via the emergency department/trauma bay
- Patients rarely arrive without emergency physician accompaniment.
- Objects are usually still in situ, which protects against active bleeding/exsanguination.

Diagnostics
- Clinical examination
  - Exploration of the foreign body (do not remove if visualization is inadequate)
  - Check peripheral pulse status
- Laboratory
  - Blood count, coagulation
- Ultrasound
  - For foreign bodies in the cervical region or extremities, good assessment of the entry site and structures around the foreign body
  - For deeper structures or pronounced soft tissue injury with hematoma, diagnostic value is greatly limited
- X-ray
  - For radiopaque objects, provides more information about size and shape
- CT angiography
  - Diagnostic tool of choice to precisely depict depth of penetration and possible associated injuries

Therapy

- Without exception, surgical
  - Preoperative preparation
  - Stabilization of the patient
  - Antibiotic therapy
  - Administration of analgesics
  - Optimization of coagulation, if necessary administration of blood transfusions/factor concentrates
  - Surgical removal in the operating room under sterile conditions
  - Carefully dissect along the object into the depth
  - Expose and, if possible, clamp injured vessels above and below
  - Then slowly remove the object
  - Depending on the extent of injury, reconstruction using patch or bypass/interposition graft may be necessary
  - Preferably use autologous (vein) or xenogeneic (bovine pericardium) material
  - Fasciotomy must be performed in case of bleeding/large soft tissue hematoma and previous ischemia
  - In case of contamination (common), do not close the wound primarily, but apply subcutaneous vacuum sealing

Call the on-call service at night?

- Yes, the foreign body must be removed promptly

Tips and Tricks

- Even if it looks very alarming: Never simply remove the object
- Ensure sufficient blood products are available for surgery
- Always disinfect and drape the surgical area extensively and prepare the leg for harvesting the great saphenous vein as needed
- Order antibiotics early

Continuation of Case Example

The wound was opened slightly under anesthesia and sterile conditions in the operating room, explored, and the stent was removed without complications and without reconstruction.

31 Avulsion of the Axillary Artery

The most common injury mechanism for traumatic lesions of the axillary artery is traumatic shoulder dislocation (Fig. 31.1) or proximal humeral fracture-dislocation. As a result, patients are almost always initially treated by trauma surgeons and then referred for consultation.

Case Example
A 53-year-old patient sustained a proximal right humerus fracture three days ago in a motorcycle accident, which was initially managed conservatively after reduction in the emergency department. However, the patient subsequently complained of increasing coldness in the right hand, and CT angiography revealed an approximately 4 cm long occlusion of the axillary artery at the level of the fracture zone. The brachial artery was filling via robust collaterals. What do you recommend?

Definition
- Trauma-induced complete transection and disruption of continuity of the axillary artery

Typical Patient
- Patient with traumatic injury to the shoulder joint or upper arm
  - Shoulder joint dislocation or
  - Shoulder joint fracture-dislocation
  - Proximal humeral head fracture

Typical On-Call Scenario
- Almost always presented via the emergency department/trauma bay
- Usually contacted by the initial treating specialty (trauma surgery)
- Occasionally a call from the OR during management of a humeral fracture with a noticeable pulse deficit

S. Regus, *Vascular Surgical Emergencies*,
https://doi.org/10.1007/978-3-662-72646-4_31

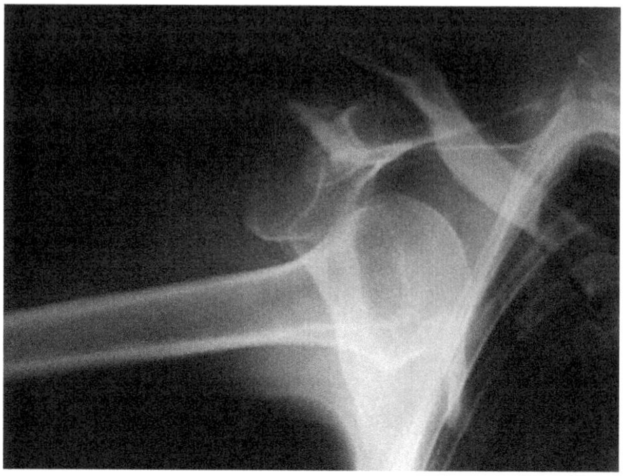

Fig. 31.1 X-ray of a patient with a shoulder joint dislocation and suspected vascular injury

- Less commonly, a consult is requested postoperatively (after initial trauma surgery management) due to abnormalities of the ipsilateral hand (coldness, sensory deficit)

Diagnostics

- Clinical examination
  - Bleeding
  - Hematoma
  - Malalignment of the shoulder joint/upper arm
  - Cool hand
  - Impaired sensorimotor function
  - No palpable pulses at the wrist or antecubital fossa
- Doppler sonography
  - of the wrist pulses using a pencil probe
  - due to swelling, wrist pulses may not be palpable but can be detected with a pencil probe
- Ultrasound
  - arterial flow signals not detectable or monophasic
  - hematoma visible in the shoulder region and upper arm
  - occasionally (rarely) visible active bleeding
- CT angiography
  - often recommended to confirm the diagnosis and, if necessary, to visualize the extent centrally

Therapy

- Conservative
  - Indications:

rarely possible
only with exceptionally good collateralization and exclusion of bleeding
- Procedure:
  Compression
  Pain management

- Interventional
  - Indications:
    in cases of incomplete vascular transection
    as bridging in emergencies
  - Procedure:
    Use of a coated (= covered) stent
- Surgical
  - Indications:
    Bleeding
    Compression symptoms
    Pain
    Ischemia
  - Procedure:
    Resection of the vessel ends
    Placement of an interposition graft
    → fundamentally autologous
    → alloplastic only in exceptional cases,
    if no vein material is available,
    but has poor patency rates and
    high risk of infection
    Exploration of the axillary vein
    → does not necessarily need to be reconstructed
    → in case of laceration, suture; otherwise, venous bleeding may occur
    after successful arterial reconstruction,
    which endangers the reconstruction outcome!
    Exploration of the axillary plexus
    → rarely injured or completely transected
    → reconstruction by nerve suture
    Fasciotomy of the forearm
    → perform if in doubt

Call the on-call service at night?
- Yes, almost always an indication for surgery

Tips and Tricks
- Critical ischemia is rare (good collateralization)
- With complete continuity injury, there is usually no active bleeding, as the vessel ends "curl up and invert"
- During exploration, always search for the proximal pulse and clamp the vessel there, then locate the site of rupture

- Always drape the thigh in a sterile manner to allow for dissection of the great saphenous vein (this is almost always suitable)
- If in doubt, perform a very generous fasciotomy, as reperfusion syndrome is often difficult to diagnose afterwards and is noticed and treated with delay.
- Often occurs at night or on weekends
- Significant risk of reconstruction occlusion due to external compression and high peripheral resistance
- High risk of amputation

Continuation of Case Example

In this case, interdisciplinary discussion of the findings and further procedure is paramount. In principle, angiography with interventional readiness would be possible. It may be "only" a local thrombosis with isolated dissection, in which case interventional thrombectomy including percutaneous transluminal angioplasty (PTA) can be successfully performed. However, if from a trauma surgery perspective an operative procedure with osteosynthesis is planned, simultaneous vascular surgical reconstruction is recommended. Due to the compensated perfusion findings, osteosynthesis could be performed first, followed by the vascular surgical procedure. If the order is reversed, there is always a risk that repositioning maneuvers will endanger the fresh vascular reconstruction. The situation is different in the stage of critical ischemia. Here, arterial reconstruction should be performed without significant delay, followed by the trauma surgical procedure.

Avulsion of the Brachial Artery

32

Avulsion of the brachial artery also most commonly occurs post-traumatically, typically following elbow dislocation or fracture-dislocations. There is usually an urgent indication for surgery, which must be organized in an interdisciplinary manner. A thigh should be draped in a sterile fashion in order to harvest the vein for use as a graft if necessary (Fig. 32.1).

Case Example
A 68-year-old, heavily intoxicated patient fell at home on the stairs and sustained a severely displaced humeral shaft fracture. The colleagues from trauma surgery notice a cold hand, and a CT angiography already performed shows an interruption of the brachial artery at the level of the fracture. Surgical management with plate osteosynthesis is planned, alternatively reduction and immobilization with an external fixator until definitive treatment. You are asked to perform the vascular exploration and, if necessary, reconstruction, and are asked when you would like to join. What is your response?

Definition

- Complete transection and disruption of continuity of the brachial artery caused by trauma

Typical Patient

- Trauma victim after elbow dislocation or fracture-dislocation
- In some cases, previous sharp force injury (e.g., stab or incised wound)
- Rare, but typical vascular lesion in children with supracondylar humerus fracture

Typical On-Call Situation

- Presentation via the emergency department/trauma bay
- Contact by the initial treating specialty (trauma surgery, pediatric surgery)

S. Regus, *Vascular Surgical Emergencies*,
https://doi.org/10.1007/978-3-662-72646-4_32

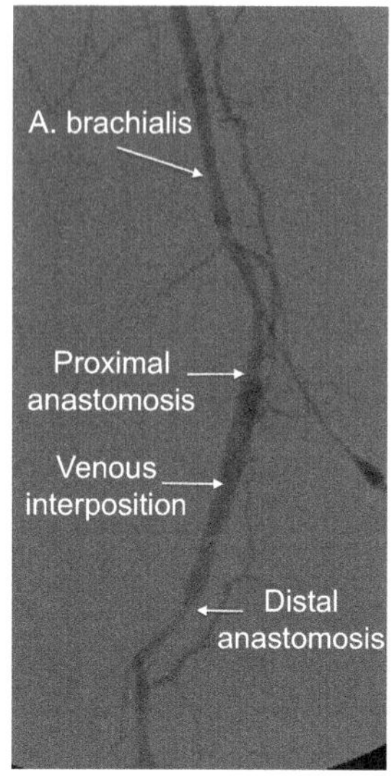

Fig. 32.1 Intraoperative angiography after reconstruction of the avulsed brachial artery with a venous interposition graft

- Occasionally a call from the OR during management of an elbow fracture with a noticeable pulse deficit
- Due to good collateralization of the brachial artery, often only noticed postoperatively
- After initial trauma surgical management, a consult request due to abnormal findings in the ipsilateral hand, such as coldness or sensory deficits
- Not infrequently, however, attributable to nerve injury

Diagnostics

- Clinical examination
  - Bleeding
  - Hematoma
  - cool hand
  - impaired sensorimotor function
  - pulses at the wrist not palpable
- Doppler sonography
  - of the wrist pulses with a pencil probe
  - Due to swelling, wrist pulses may not be palpable but can be detected with a pencil probe.
- Ultrasound
  - arterial flow signals
  - hematoma
  - visible active bleeding
- CT angiography
  - indicated only in exceptional cases

Therapy

- Conservative
  - Indications:
    rarely possible
    in cases of local dissection without disruption of continuity
  - Approach:
    heparin infusion or therapeutic LMWH
    pain management
- Interventional
  - Indications:
    in short-segment dissection with intraluminal thrombosis
    in active bleeding and inoperability
  - Approach:
    aspiration
    lysis
    covered stent (usually as bridging prior to surgical management)
- Surgical
  - Indications:
    active spurting bleeding
    acute ischemia Rutherford IIb
    compartment syndrome
  - Approach:
    treatment of choice
    exploration of the artery
    thrombectomy, suture or reconstruction (interposition graft from the great saphenous vein)
    fasciotomy, if necessary with VAC dressing

Call the on-call consultant at night?

- Yes, usually an indication for surgery

Tips and Tricks

- Surgical intervention should be preferred
- Even in cases of complete loss of continuity, bleeding is usually minor, as the vessel ends tend to retract
- Before completing the suture and releasing blood flow, always check for good peripheral backflow to rule out prior embolization and, if necessary, perform a thrombectomy
- Wash and drape the thigh in a sterile manner to allow harvesting of the great saphenous vein
- During or after successful lysis treatment, it may become apparent that there was indeed a vessel wall lesion, which had been masked by the thrombus. Therefore, the risk of bleeding is very high afterwards

- Close monitoring is essential!
- Indicate fasciotomy in a timely manner

Case Example Continued

You request the earliest possible trauma surgery intervention with repositioning and application of an external fixator, so that vascular exploration can be performed without significant delay (preferably simultaneously). You also request that the arm be placed on an "arm table" and that one leg be draped in a sterile manner in case the great saphenous vein needs to be harvested. Ideally, you should be present in the operating room during positioning and inform the on-call senior physician in good time.

Avulsion of the Popliteal Artery

33

Avulsion of the popliteal artery is a typical complication following severe knee joint trauma (Fig. 33.1), but is usually well compensated and asymptomatic initially due to good collateral circulation. For this reason, a pulse deficit of the popliteal artery is often only noticed during orthopedic trauma surgery.

Case Example
You receive a call from the trauma surgery OR, where a patient with a complex knee injury following dislocation is currently being treated. There is massive bleeding in the popliteal fossa, and you are asked to take a look. Upon exploration, you see oozing bleeding in the popliteal fossa. The patient is in the prone position. What do you do to confirm or rule out suspicion of injury to the popliteal artery?

Definition

- Traumatic injury and disruption of continuity of the popliteal artery

Typical Patient

- Trauma surgery patient with knee dislocation/dislocation fracture (blunt injury)
- More common in men, ratio m:f = 9:1
- Less commonly, sharp transection of the popliteal artery (stab wound)
- In children, occasionally laceration from broken glass after a fall

Typical On-Call Situation

- Contact from trauma surgery due to a "cold leg" after knee trauma
- Sometimes also a call from the OR because the vessel cannot be visualized or there is uncontrolled bleeding

S. Regus, *Vascular Surgical Emergencies*,
https://doi.org/10.1007/978-3-662-72646-4_33

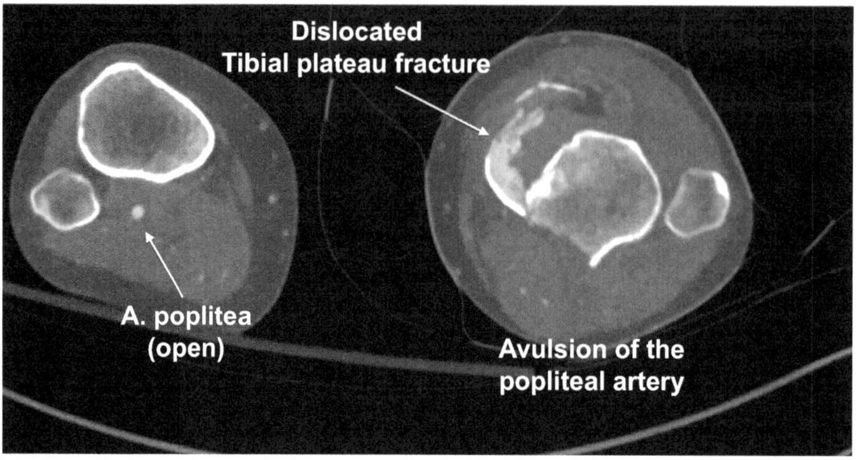

Fig. 33.1 CTA of a patient after knee dislocation with displaced tibial fracture and avulsion of the popliteal artery

Diagnostics

- Inspection
  - Hematoma, swelling
  - dusky discoloration of foot/toes
- Examination
  - Pulse status is extremely important
  - Sensory disturbances may also be due to tibial nerve injury
  - Temperature difference between sides may be a clue, but is by no means definitive
    may also be due to clothing injury, inadequate body covering, or prolonged lying outdoors
- Ultrasound
  - difficult, as there is often a large hematoma
  - Doppler sonographic assessment of foot pulses can be very helpful, especially in the OR
- CT angiography
  - Diagnostic tool of choice
- Angiography (DSA)
  - not indicated as initial diagnostic
  - only if CT is not available or
  - if emergency intervention is planned
    Angiography with interventional readiness

Therapy

- Conservative
  - Indications:

In cases of short-segment dissection without occlusion, a conservative therapeutic attempt can be made.
However, a vascular wall lesion with active bleeding must be ruled out.
  - Approach:
    Heparin administration via perfusor
    if necessary, gentle wrapping of the arm
    Cooling, elevation, rest
    Pain management
- Interventional
  - Indications:
    partial tear
    dissection with occlusion
  - Approach:
    Lysis
    Aspiration
    Implantation of a coated stent
    Interventional procedures are rarely promising at this location (mobile segment), but may be used as a bridge for bleeding control.
- Surgical
  - Indications:
    complete transection
    active bleeding
    critical ischemia
    compartment syndrome
  - Approach:
    Suturing
    Reconstruction by end-to-end anastomosis
    Patch angioplasty
    Interposition graft for longer defects (ideally with a bovine patch or autologous vein)
    Hematoma evacuation
    Fasciotomy

Call the on-call consultant at night?
- Yes, usually an indication for surgery

Tips and Tricks
- If the patient has palpable foot pulses, a popliteal artery rupture can be virtually ruled out (but caution: sometimes you may be feeling your own pulse)
- Doppler sonographic visualization of the foot pulses as an exclusion method (especially in the OR under sterile conditions) is very helpful, but less suitable for confirming the diagnosis
- A missing signal may also be due to a lack of ultrasound gel or device malfunction

- No false "cosmetic concerns": fasciotomy (even prophylactically) can save the limb
- DSA with interventional readiness should only be performed after prior CTA to allow for possible percutaneous transluminal angioplasty (PTA)/lysis

Case Study Continuation

You ask the nurse (circulating nurse in the OR) to arrange for a Doppler probe and have it covered in a sterile manner. With this, you can attempt to detect arterial signals at the foot. If this is successful, suturing the bleeding source would be recommended. However, if you are unable to detect foot pulses and the artery cannot be found in the surgical field, angiography would be a helpful diagnostic tool. For this, the patient would need to be placed in the supine position and the angiography performed via the groin. If it is indeed a rupture of the popliteal artery and it cannot be visualized via the dorsal approach, reconstruction will generally need to be performed via a supra- and infragenual approach in the supine position anyway.

Part IX
Supra-aortic Arterial Diseases

Symptomatic Carotid Stenosis

34

Symptomatic carotid stenosis (Fig. 34.1) is a common reason for the stroke unit to contact vascular surgery on call, but an emergency surgical indication is rarely present.

Case Example

A general practitioner refers a 63-year-old female patient for "emergency" surgery with the suspected diagnosis of symptomatic carotid stenosis. The patient reports that she has repeatedly experienced dizziness for several weeks, especially when moving from a sitting to a standing position. She denies any specific neurological deficits such as arm weakness or unilateral visual disturbances. She has not had a stroke so far, but did have a heart attack three years ago, which was treated with a stent. Sonography reveals an approximately 50% stenosis of the right internal carotid artery (ICA) near its origin; the left side appears unremarkable and free of stenosis. What do you suggest?

Definition

- Stenosis of the ICA, rarely of the common carotid artery (CCA), causing cerebral ischemic symptoms

Typical Patient

- Older patient > 60 years, rarely younger
- Cardiovascular risk profile
- Often already known carotid stenosis, previously asymptomatic and (ideally) under regular surveillance

Typical On-Call Situation

- Patients are often referred for surgical evaluation by neurology for consultation
- Sometimes also referred to outpatient clinic by general practitioner/specialist

S. Regus, *Vascular Surgical Emergencies*,
https://doi.org/10.1007/978-3-662-72646-4_34

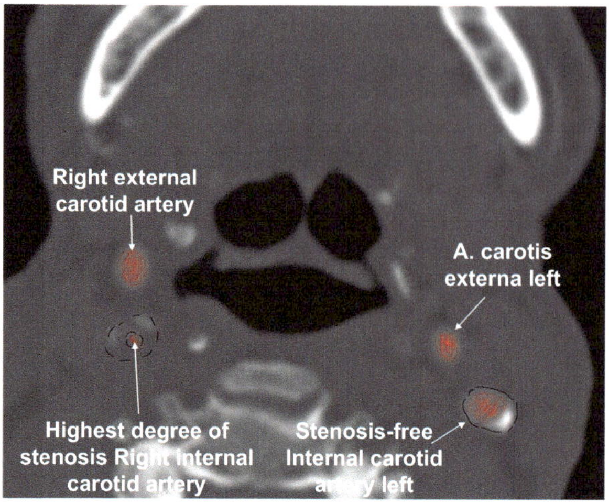

Fig. 34.1 CTA of a high-grade symptomatic stenosis of the right internal carotid artery with a soft plaque (appearing dark on CTA). A hard plaque appears bright or white.

Diagnostics

- Medical history
  - known carotid stenosis?
  - history of surgery or stent?
- Clinical examination
  - Signs of symptomatic carotid stenosis
    contralateral peripheral hemisymptoms
      $\rightarrow$usually arm-predominant (coffee cup falls from hand)
    transient visual disturbances = ipsilateral amaurosis fugax
    Speech and word-finding disturbances
      $\rightarrow$reported by relatives
      $\rightarrow$The speech center is located in the dominant hemisphere, i.e., on the left in right-handed individuals and on the right in left-handed individuals.
      $\rightarrow$A high-grade left ICA stenosis with speech disturbances is considered symptomatic ICA stenosis in right-handed individuals, but asymptomatic in left-handed individuals.
- Sonography
  - Stenosis?
  - hard or soft plaques?
  - Degree of stenosis?
  - Occlusion?
- CT angiography
  - Visualization of the stenosis
  - Characterization of the occlusion (soft or hard plaque)
  - Visualization of central outflow
  - intracranial visualization

- MRA
  - as an alternative to CTA
  - in case of contrast agent allergy or
  - young women of childbearing age
  - Disadvantages:
    takes longer
    poorer assessment of vessel wall and plaque
    stenoses are often "overestimated"

Therapy

- Conservative
  - Indications:
    for mild stenosis < 50%
    if disabling stroke (from Rankin 3)
  - Approach:
    BMT
      → Antihypertensives
      → Antiplatelet therapy
      → Statins
    initially aim for rehabilitation and re-evaluate at follow-up clinic visits
- Interventional
  - Indications:
    ≥50% symptomatic stenosis
    acute long-segment occlusion
    stenoses at the skull base or intracranially
  - Approach:
    Stent-PTA as an alternative to surgical reconstruction is possible
    Thrombolysis and, if necessary, intervention in case of a fresh occlusion extending intracranially
    neuroradiological intervention intracranially
- Surgical
  - Indications:
    ≥50% symptomatic stenosis
    long-segment soft plaque
    Crescendo TIA (recurrent TIAs with progressive symptoms)
      → Emergency indication!
  - Approach:
    Carotid endarterectomy (CEA) with patch angioplasty
    Eversion endarterectomy (EEA)
    with neuromonitoring

Call the on-call service at night?

- When in doubt, always call in carotid emergencies
- Mandatory in case of worsening symptoms or acute occlusion to discuss further management

Tips and Tricks

- For symptomatic stenosis with an indication for intervention or surgery, this should be performed as soon as possible, within 14 days
- Try to obtain two imaging studies (usually sonography and CTA)
- Stay calm; an emergency indication is extremely rare and excessive intervention increases the risk of complications
  - There are two emergency indications:
    acute thrombotic occlusion of the carotid bifurcation
    Crescendo TIA (TIAs at short intervals with increasing neurological deficits)
- Always examine the patient clinically and assess the situation. If the condition is extremely poor, critically evaluate the indication for surgery and consider rehabilitation first
- If symptoms occurred more than 6 months ago, the stenosis is, by definition, asymptomatic
- Dizziness is not a typical sign!!
- In patients with previous surgery or radiation, many prefer stent-PTA, but surgery is also possible in principle

Case Example Continued

Since the patient does not present with any specific neurological deficits suggestive of a middle cerebral artery ischemia (dizziness is not a typical symptom), this is, by definition, an asymptomatic moderate-grade origin stenosis of the right ICA. There is no indication for surgery in this case. A sonographic follow-up in 3–6 months and "Best Medical Treatment" are recommended. In addition, referral to cardiology and, if necessary, neurology would be indicated to further clarify the dizziness. Both can be managed on an outpatient basis; inpatient admission is not indicated if vital parameters are unremarkable.

35 Acute Carotid Occlusion

Acute symptomatic occlusion of the internal carotid artery (Fig. 35.1)—alongside symptomatic carotid stenosis with crescendo TIA—constitutes an emergency indication for invasive revascularization via stent PTA or surgery.

Case Example

The on-call neurologist from the stroke unit contacts you and requests an assessment of a 67-year-old patient who was admitted for a high-grade, 90% symptomatic right-sided ICA stenosis. The patient is now exhibiting fluctuating neurological deficits with ipsilateral visual disturbances in the form of amaurosis fugax. The deficits are progressive and the intervals between episodes are becoming shorter. In addition, current sonography reveals an acute occlusion of the previously described high-grade stenosis. Do you wait until the next day or contact your on-call backup?

Definition

- Acute occlusion of the carotid arteries
- Usually located at the carotid bifurcation and sometimes extending intracerebrally

Typical Patient

- A typical "vascular patient" with a cardiovascular risk profile and known atherosclerosis
- However, acute (usually embolic) carotid occlusion can also occur in patients without vascular disease.
- Ultimately, traumatic occlusion can also occur, in this case due to dissection or a blunt (hyperextension trauma) or sharp (stab, puncture, gunshot wound) lesion.

S. Regus, *Vascular Surgical Emergencies*,
https://doi.org/10.1007/978-3-662-72646-4_35

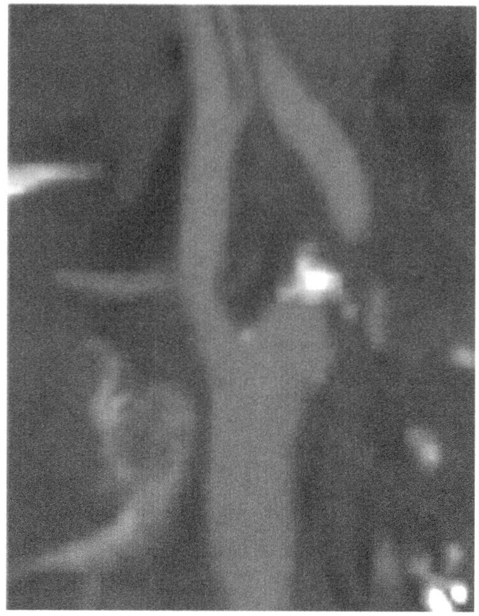

Fig. 35.1 CTA (sagittal slice) shows an acute carotid occlusion

Typical On-Call Scenario

- Rarely is the patient presented directly to vascular surgery.
- Most often, the patient is referred for consultation from the stroke unit, where they were initially admitted
- But sometimes also from cardiology, in patients with arrhythmias and emboli
- Rarely from one's own department, e.g., patients with previous limb ischemia due to embolism, who then subsequently suffer an "upward" embolism into the territory of the carotid artery

Diagnostics

- Clinical examination
  - Signs of previous TIA or
  - Assessment of cerebral damage using the Rankin Scale 0–6
    0: no symptoms
    1: not relevant
    2: independent without aids
    3: independent with aids
    4: unable to walk or stand
    5: bedridden, incontinent
    6: death
- Sonography
  - the initial and often already diagnostic procedure

- CT angiography
  - for diagnostic confirmation and therapy planning
  - plaque morphology and vessel wall can be well assessed
- MRA
  - also possible as an alternative
  - however, vessel wall and characteristics of the occlusion are often insufficiently assessable here
- CCT or MRI of the brain
  - should always be performed to visualize the cerebral situation and establish a baseline
  - a fulminant infarct with midline shift is often a contraindication for further invasive measures

Therapy

- Conservative
  - Indications:
    if a supposedly acute occlusion appears chronic (calcified) on CTA
    in the case of a disabling infarct (Rankin 5)
    →palliative treatment
    in the case of a large infarct
    →risk of hemorrhage
  - Procedure:
    heparin infusion
    pain management
    if necessary, rehabilitation and subsequent reevaluation
- Interventional
  - Indications:
    nowadays, the majority of acute thrombotic occlusions
    Exclusion of contraindications:
    →bleeding
    →cerebral malignancy/metastases
    →major visceral, trauma, or carotid surgery within the last 14 days
  - Procedure:
    local or systemic thrombolysis
    stent PTA
    if stenoses are unmasked
- Surgical
  - Indications:
    acute occlusion of the ICA at its origin with underlying high-grade stenosis
    contraindications for thrombolysis
  - Procedure:
    thromboendarterectomy (TEA) with patch plasty
    →in some cases, outflow must also be thrombectomized

Call the on-call service at night?

- Contact is almost always recommended

Tips and Tricks

- CTA as the diagnostic tool of choice:
  - Sometimes a supposedly acute carotid occlusion is actually chronic and cannot be surgically recanalized
  - In CTA, fresh and old occlusions can be well distinguished from each other
  - This is less reliable in MRA
- Be cautious of clinical deterioration after surgery/thrombolysis, as this may be caused by reperfusion of a large infarct area
- A hypertensive crisis postoperatively or post-interventionally can be fatal due to cerebral hemorrhage and should be strictly avoided
- A carotid occlusion can often be asymptomatic in the presence of pre-existing stenosis. However, these patients do not usually present as emergencies, so the diagnosis of carotid occlusion is often made only during follow-up duplex sonographic examinations

Continuation of Case Example

As a general rule, it is advisable to contact the on-call service very liberally in the event of complications and problems in the carotid circulation. Especially in the case of a crescendo TIA, as described here, or in acute carotid occlusion (and even more so if both are present), emergency surgical intervention is indicated and contacting the on-call service is absolutely essential. Under no circumstances should you wait until the next day.

36 Acute Carotid Dissection

Acute carotid dissection is a vascular disease that can be managed conservatively, usually occurring spontaneously or as a result of a hypertensive crisis in the presence of pre-existing atherosclerosis. However, cervical spine trauma can also be a cause of dissection of the cervical vessels. In cases of aortic dissection, it is standard practice to also examine the carotid arteries.

Case Example
A 36-year-old female patient is admitted to the emergency department following a suicide attempt by hanging. She is intubated and ventilated, has no bony injuries, but CT reveals a short-segment dissection of the internal carotid artery (ICA) near the origin on both sides. There is no evidence of intracerebral hemorrhage or ischemia, and the ICA above the dissection is unremarkably perfused on both sides. The trauma surgery colleagues ask whether stent implantation is necessary. What is your response? (Fig. 36.1)

Definition
- Dissection of the carotid artery, often the common and/or internal carotid artery
- But also possible at the skull base
- Sometimes extending intracranially
- Mostly traumatic, rarely spontaneous
- Occasionally also occurs in the context of an aortic dissection (Stanford A)

Typical Patient
- Younger patient after a traffic accident (cervical spine trauma)
- Suicide attempt by hanging
- External violence by (manual) strangulation
- Older patient with a cardiovascular risk profile
- Patient in a stroke unit after cerebral infarction and suspected dissection on sonography or CT angiography

S. Regus, *Vascular Surgical Emergencies*,
https://doi.org/10.1007/978-3-662-72646-4_36

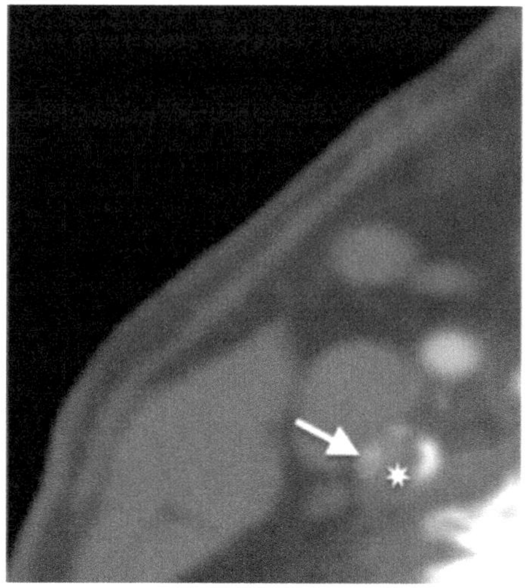

Fig. 36.1 CTA of an acute dissection of the internal carotid artery with thrombosis of the false lumen (asterisk) and compression of the true lumen (arrow)

Typical On-Call Situation
- Overall very rare in vascular surgery on-call service
- Polytraumatized patient with cervical spine involvement in the emergency department
- Consultation from the stroke unit with suspected dissection on sonography or "incidental finding" on CT angiography
- Consultation for a patient (usually cardiology) with hypertensive crisis and neurological abnormalities

Diagnostics
- Clinical examination
  - basic neurological assessment
  - contusions, strangulation marks, or wounds post-trauma
  - signs of middle cerebral artery ischemia
  - headache, nausea
  - possibly ipsilateral Horner's syndrome
- Duplex sonography
  - for orientation
- CT angiography
  - in suspected carotid dissection, regardless of underlying etiology, the diagnostic method of choice

Therapy
- Conservative
  - Indications:
    most commonly used
    for uncomplicated dissection without significant associated injuries
    short-segment findings without bleeding/perforation

- Approach:
  strict blood pressure control
  antiplatelet therapy
  anticoagulation only in case of occlusion or pseudo-occlusion
- Interventional
  - Indications:
    in acute thrombotic occlusion and
    corresponding neurological deficit
  - Approach:
    systemic or local thrombolysis with rtPA (Actilyse®)
    stent angioplasty
- Surgical
  - Indications:
    in Stanford type A dissection → cardiac surgery
    in case of bleeding/perforation
    in thrombotic occlusion of the carotid bifurcation
    in intracranial hemorrhage and contraindication to thrombolysis
    after unsuccessful intervention
  - Approach:
    very rarely indicated due to high risk of complications
    thrombectomy and patch or interposition graft
    fixation of the distal intimal flap is extremely important

Call the on-call consultant at night?
- If there is an acute carotid occlusion with cerebral infarction, active bleeding, or Stanford type A dissection, to discuss further therapeutic management

Tips and Tricks
- Diagnosis is often difficult because symptoms are nonspecific
- Horner's syndrome (ptosis, miosis, enophthalmos) due to injury of the sympathetic trunk or stellate ganglion (running posterior to the ICA)
- Occurs spontaneously (usually hypertensive crisis) or can also be traumatic
- There is insufficient evidence as to whether oral anticoagulation is beneficial
- Antiplatelet therapy is usually sufficient, duration at least 6 months, lifelong in the case of atherosclerosis
- Surgical indication is rare and should always be considered critically, as the procedure is technically quite demanding and prone to complications (in particular, the distal end is sometimes difficult to expose and control)
- Intervention (lysis, PTA, stent) may be considered in cases of acute cerebral ischemic symptoms

Case Example Continued

Stent implantation is not indicated; the treatment of choice is purely conservative. A CCT follow-up after 6 hours is recommended to rule out a demarcating ischemia. In addition, a follow-up CTA of the carotids in 24–48 hours is advisable. Depending on concomitant injuries, administration of unfractionated heparin at a therapeutic dose is indicated; blood pressure spikes should be avoided.

Part X
Diseases of the Abdominal and Pelvic Arteries

37 Ruptured Abdominal Aortic Aneurysm (rAAA)

The ruptured aortic aneurysm (Fig. 37.1) is **the emergency** in vascular surgery par excellence, and the one most feared at the beginning of training. The typical symptom triad consists of abdominal/lumbar pain, a pulsating mass, and collapse.

Case Example
You receive a call from a colleague at a nearby smaller hospital requesting transfer of a patient with a ruptured aortic aneurysm, as they do not have a vascular surgeon. You want to know a bit more about the patient and learn that it is an 89-year-old patient with a long-standing known abdominal aortic aneurysm. Current CT imaging shows a contained rupture with a maximum diameter of 11 cm. The patient is responsive and hemodynamically stable. Is there anything you should absolutely clarify before transfer?

Definition
- Tear in the wall of an aortic aneurysm
- An aortic aneurysm is defined as a diameter of approximately 3 cm or more.
- Contained rupture: into the retroperitoneum (i.e., posteriorly)
- Free rupture: into the abdominal cavity or thorax, usually resulting in "sudden cardiac death" or "death from exsanguination"

Typical Patient
- Usually older patient with cardiovascular risk factors and known aortic aneurysm
- Smokers may be affected even in middle age
- Rarely younger patients (Marfan, Ehlers-Danlos, Loeys-Dietz syndrome)

Typical On-Call Situation
- Often a dramatic announcement in the emergency department
- Hemodynamically unstable patient with abdominal and/or back pain

S. Regus, *Vascular Surgical Emergencies*,
https://doi.org/10.1007/978-3-662-72646-4_37

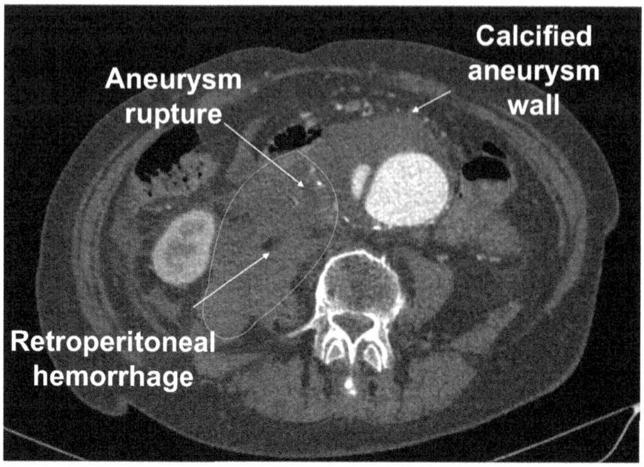

Fig. 37.1 CTA of a ruptured abdominal aortic aneurysm (rAAA) with retroperitoneal hemorrhage

- Rarely (but not to be underestimated) a less dramatic patient who "walks" into the emergency department with only abdominal or lumbar pain (if retroperitoneal bleeding is well tamponaded)

Diagnostics
- Often already a history of known aortic aneurysm
- Triad is key:
  - abdominal pain
  - pulsating swelling
  - collapse
- Focused ultrasound in the trauma bay
- If the patient is stable, then CT angiography
- If the patient is unstable, take directly to the OR without further diagnostics (any delay costs time)

Therapy
- Conservative
  - Indications:
    malignant underlying disease
    refusal of surgery (often already in the asymptomatic stage during follow-up)
    inoperability
  - Approach:
    Pain management with morphine infusion (1–2 mg/h)
    Placement in a single room (for reasons of dignity!)

- Interventional
  - Indications:
    if treatment is desired and
    if suitable morphology
  - Approach:
    if necessary, REBOA ("resuscitative endovascular balloon occlusion of the aorta") maneuver, which can be performed in unstable patients already in the trauma bay
    endovascular exclusion
    → aortobiiliac (if a selection of prostheses is available on site) or
    → aortomonoiliac and crossover bypass
- Open surgical
  - Indications:
    if endovascular treatment is not possible
    → unsuitable morphology
    → no prostheses available on site
  - Approach:
    crossmatch 6 units of packed red blood cells!!!
    median laparotomy or retroperitoneal approach
    aortobiiliac Y-graft (14–7 for women and 16–8 for men) or
    aortic tube graft (14/16/18/20)

Call the on-call consultant at night?
- Emergency indication
- If the patient refuses surgery, admit for palliative care (morphine infusion) and inform the consultant the following day
- Under resuscitation conditions, surgical therapy is usually not promising, but it is still advisable to inform the on-call consultant

Tips and Tricks
- Ask anesthesia to only induce in the operating room once the patient has been prepped in a sterile manner and the surgical team is at the table. Otherwise, muscle relaxation can compromise the retroperitoneal tamponade, which may lead to patient instability.
- For stable patients, aim for a CTA, especially if endovascular treatment is planned.
- For unstable patients, do not delay by performing a CTA.
- If endovascular therapy is indicated but suitable prosthetic material is not available, aorto-monoiliac repair is possible with subsequent crossover bypass.

Case Example Continued
It is important to know why the patient, despite having a known and such a large aortic aneurysm, did not undergo elective surgery beforehand. Often, patients

consciously decide against surgery and do not wish to have it even in the event of a rupture. You should therefore explicitly ask whether the patient wants surgery. If the patient declines, you can spare them the stress of being transported to your hospital, only for them to personally inform you on site of their refusal of the surgical procedure.

Ruptured Iliac Aneurysm (rIA) 38

A ruptured iliac aneurysm is a rare but highly lethal vascular surgical emergency. Typically, initial presentation is to urology. However, the suspected diagnosis of a ureteral colic can usually be quickly ruled out, and suspicion of an aneurysm rupture is raised.

Case Example
The on-call urologist contacts you regarding a patient who was referred to him with the suspected diagnosis of a right-sided ureteral colic. However, sonography raised suspicion that the patient has an iliac aneurysm, and the ureter is free of stones. The patient is currently asymptomatic, hemodynamically stable, and has a hemoglobin value of 16.2 g/dl. The abdominal wall is soft, with mild tenderness and guarding in the right lower abdomen. What is your recommendation? (Fig. 38.1)

Definition
- Ruptured aneurysm of the iliac artery
- Rarely isolated (approx. 3–5%), usually occurs together with an aortic aneurysm (approx. 95–98%)

Typical Patient
- Middle-aged to older adults
- Men >> women
- The common iliac artery is most frequently affected, followed by the internal iliac artery
- Most often on the right
- Symptoms similar to ruptured aortic aneurysm:
  - Abdominal/back pain
  - possibly radiating to the groin

S. Regus, *Vascular Surgical Emergencies*,
https://doi.org/10.1007/978-3-662-72646-4_38

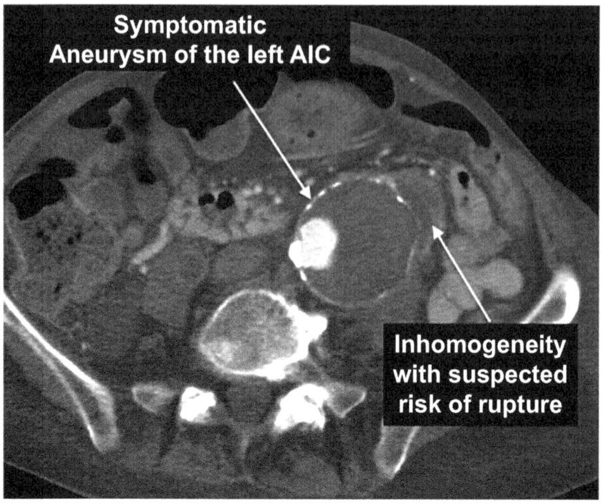

Fig. 38.1 CTA of a symptomatic aneurysm of the left common iliac artery (D_{max} 5.5 cm), which was urgently treated due to presumed risk of rupture

  - tender abdomen on palpation
  - rigid abdominal wall
  - shock
- Typical patient with a cardiovascular risk profile
- Rarely genetic disorders (Marfan syndrome, Loeys-Dietz syndrome, Ehlers-Danlos syndrome)

Typical On-Call Situation

- Via emergency department with acute abdominal pain
- Typically also referred for consultation from urology with flank and groin pain
- Often more stable than patients with ruptured aortic aneurysm due to contained rupture
- Usually at night or in the early morning hours (blood pressure rise after going to the bathroom)

Diagnostics

- Clinical examination
  - watch for the triad:
    abdominal pain (acute abdomen)
    pulsatile mass
    shock
- Laboratory and blood gas analysis
  - Hemoglobin! Already in the ambulance, at the latest in the emergency department

- Sonography
  - for orientation
  - often in the trauma bay
- CT angiography
  - if suspicion of ruptured iliac aneurysm and
  - patient is stable!
  - if patient is unstable, no further diagnostics and proceed to emergency surgery

Therapy

- Conservative
  - Indications:
    In principle, there is an indication for emergency surgery!
    However, even here, the patient's condition, their wishes, and chances of survival must be taken into account.
    In unstable patients under resuscitation conditions, the chances of survival are extremely low, so the indication for surgery should be critically questioned and clarified with relatives.
    Some patients have already declined elective surgery in advance when an aneurysm was known. This patient preference should also be respected in emergency situations.
  - Procedure:
    Pain management using a morphine infusion pump (1–2 mg/h)
    single room accommodation if possible!
- Interventional (endovascular)
  - Indications or prerequisites:
    Morphology with a sufficiently long landing zone
    suitable prostheses available on site
    expertise and equipment (hybrid operating room)
  - Procedure:
    Implantation of an aortoiliac stent graft
    sometimes also as a Y-graft bi-iliac
    if necessary, closure of the IIA
- Open surgical
  - Indications:
    hemorrhagic shock
    large retroperitoneal hematoma requiring decompression
    no suitable prosthetic material available on site
    unsuccessful endovascular treatment attempt
    → so-called conversion surgery
    In principle, any ruptured or symptomatic iliac aneurysm can also be treated with open surgery.
  - Procedure:
    for clarity, a midline laparotomy is preferred
    placement of an iliac interposition graft
    if necessary, aortobiiliac interposition required

Call the on-call service at night?

- Emergency surgery is indicated, so it is essential to contact the on-call team

Tips and Tricks

- Ultrasound as the first diagnostic tool
  - Aneurysm is usually located on the right in the common iliac artery
- CTA only in stable patients or—if possible—directly in the operating room
- Open surgery is always technically possible
  - but keep the operative time as short as possible
  - no aortobiiliac reconstruction in moderately stable patients if there are other intact and electively non-treatable aortic aneurysms (<5.5 cm) or contralateral iliac aneurysms (<3.5 cm)
- Endovascular often as aortobiiliac prosthesis or aortomonoiliac with prior exclusion of the IIA (coils, occluder)
  - but then a crossover bypass is still necessary

Continuation of Case Study

Based on the findings, the likelihood of rupture of the iliac aneurysm is unlikely; nevertheless, you should perform a CTA to rule this out. If the aneurysm is confirmed and there is no rupture, it should be classified as a symptomatic aneurysm and inpatient monitoring is strongly recommended. Systolic blood pressure should not exceed 140 mmHg, ideally remaining at 120/80 mmHg. Invasive treatment would be indicated for a symptomatic aneurysm regardless of the maximum diameter and should be performed early-electively on the next, or at the latest the following, regular working day. The type of treatment—open or endovascular—depends on the morphology and internal clinical standards.

Acute Aortic Dissection

39

In clinical practice, acute aortic dissection is classified according to Stanford as type A and B, the latter further divided into uncomplicated (Fig. 39.1) or complicated (with instability or organ malperfusion). The "B dissection" falls under the domain of vascular surgery, while the "A dissection" is managed by cardiac surgeons.

Case Example

You need to inform a 58-year-old patient with an acute complicated type B aortic dissection, who is experiencing visceral and renal malperfusion, about the endovascular procedure (TEVAR). He is very anxious and asks you about possible complications, especially the risk of paraplegia. What do you tell him?

Definition

- Acute tear of the aortic wall layers between the intima and adventitia, located in the media layer
- Classification by time course:
  - acute: <14 days
  - subacute: 14–90 days
  - chronic: >90 days
- Classification by body region:
  - thoracic (approx. 90%)
  - less commonly abdominal (approx. 10%)
- Classification by location:
  - according to Stanford:
    A: Ascending aorta (originating before the left subclavian artery)
    B: Descending aorta (originating distal to the left subclavian artery)
    →uncomplicated
    Pain symptoms mild to moderate

S. Regus, *Vascular Surgical Emergencies*,
https://doi.org/10.1007/978-3-662-72646-4_39

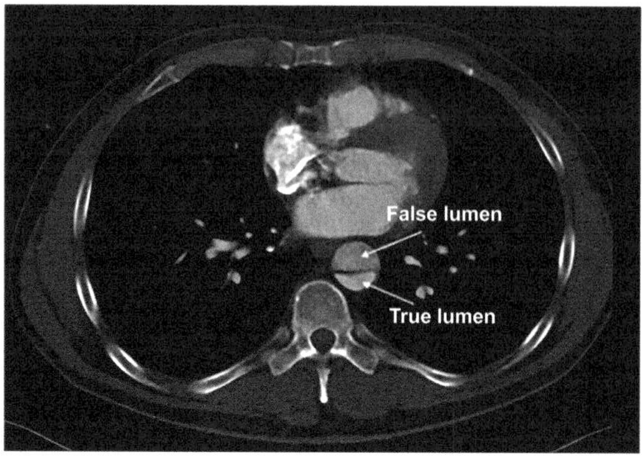

Fig. 39.1 CTA of an uncomplicated Stanford type B aortic dissection

Renal or visceral vessels not involved
← complicated
progressive, severe pain
with occlusion of renal or visceral vessels

– according to DeBakey:
  I: originating in the ascending aorta, distal extent unlimited
  II: confined to the ascending aorta, aortic arch and descending aorta are free
  III: originating in the descending aorta after the left subclavian artery branches off
    IIIa: distal end above the diaphragm (thus limited to the thoracic aorta)
    IIIb: distal end below the diaphragm (abdominal aorta also involved)

Typical Patient

- More common in men
- Age 50–70
- Typically known arterial hypertension
- Obesity
- Smoker
- Stress (managers, executives, often still employed)

Typical On-Call Situation

- Usually via the emergency department
- Often initially seen in cardiology with suspected myocardial infarction
- Sometimes also as a consult from cardiology or the intensive care unit
- Typically also from the "cardiac catheterization lab" if the cardiac catheterization is unremarkable and dissection is noted on echocardiography
- Emergency presentation to internal medicine due to a hypertensive crisis/emergency

Diagnostics

- Laboratory
  - often markedly elevated D-dimers are notable
- Ultrasound
  - Transthoracic (TTE) or transesophageal (TEE) echocardiography
  - Dissection membrane visible in the ascending aorta and sometimes the arch
  - Descending aorta usually not assessable
- CT angiography
  - preferred advanced diagnostic method
  - fast
  - wall and lumen well assessable
  - extent clearly visible

Therapy

- Conservative
  - Indications:
    uncomplicated type B dissection
    complicated type B or type A dissection, but
      →inoperability
      →patient preference (refusal of invasive procedures)
  - Approach:
    antihypertensive therapy
    if necessary, anticoagulation
    CTA monitoring (not in cases of inoperability, as it has no consequence)
- Interventional/endovascular
  - Indications:
    complicated type B dissection
    progression on follow-up
    cerebral stroke
    peripheral ischemia involving the extremity arteries
    type A dissection (including retrograde)
  - Approach:
    TEVAR in suitable morphology
- Surgical
  - Indications:
    complicated type B dissection after unsuccessful intervention
    type A dissection (including retrograde)
    cerebral and central complications
  - Approach:
    emergency presentation/transfer to cardiac surgery for further management of type A dissection
    peripheral or cervical/cerebral thrombectomy
    femoral/viscerorenal reconstruction

Call the on-call service at night?

- Uncomplicated type B dissection: admit to intensive care unit and inform the next morning
- Complicated type B dissection: call
- Type A dissection: emergency transfer to cardiac surgery

Tips and Tricks

- The Stanford classification is simpler and has become established in clinical practice.
  - Mnemonic: A = begins in the ascending aorta, B = "beyond brachiocephalic vessels"

- Even an uncomplicated type B dissection can become dangerous due to complications, especially a retrograde type A dissection.
- Therefore, even conservatively managed uncomplicated type B dissections should always be monitored in an intensive care setting.
- For TEVAR, treating the proximal entry with a 15–20 mm long stent graft is often sufficient, which can be easily extended if necessary.
- The longer the stent graft, the greater the risk of spinal ischemia due to occlusion of the artery of Adamkiewicz (A. radicularis magna).
  - Risk can be up to 20% if the entire thoracic aorta is treated with a stent

Case Example Continued

The risk of paraplegia depends on the length of the aortic pathology and the implanted stent graft. In particular, long-segment stent grafts are associated with an increased risk of paraplegia, which can be as high as 20%. The most important spinal cord artery (A. radicularis magna, "artery of Adamkiewicz") cannot yet be reliably visualized or protected; effective measures include maintaining a high-normal blood pressure (systolic usually at least 140 mmHg) and controlling cerebrospinal fluid pressure with target values of a maximum of 7 mmHg.

40 Leriche Syndrome

Leriche syndrome is usually acute and is considered a life-threatening aortic emergency. However, there is also a chronic Leriche syndrome (Fig. 40.1), which is well compensated and typically becomes clinically symptomatic through thigh pain or even impotence.

Case Example

A 72-year-old female patient is admitted as an emergency due to acute ischemia in both legs. Examination reveals cool lower extremities bilaterally with reduced sensorimotor function. No pulses are palpable in either leg, not even in the groin. The patient is in sinus rhythm, and sonography raises suspicion of an aortic occlusion. The creatinine level is elevated at 3.2 mg/dl due to known chronic renal insufficiency. The radiologist asks whether an MRA can be performed instead of the requested CTA, as he fears worsening of the renal insufficiency. He could arrange for an immediate MRA. What is your response?

Definition

- Occlusion of the aorta including the aortic bifurcation and the pelvic arteries
- Acute (within 14 days) or chronic (> 14 days)

Typical Patient

- Frequently smokers
- Older patients with cardiac arrhythmias
- Status post aortoiliac vascular interventions (often stent PTA)
- Known (or as yet undiagnosed) underlying malignant disease

Typical On-Call Situation

- Presentation to the emergency department with acute pain and a sensation of cold in both legs

S. Regus, *Vascular Surgical Emergencies*,
https://doi.org/10.1007/978-3-662-72646-4_40

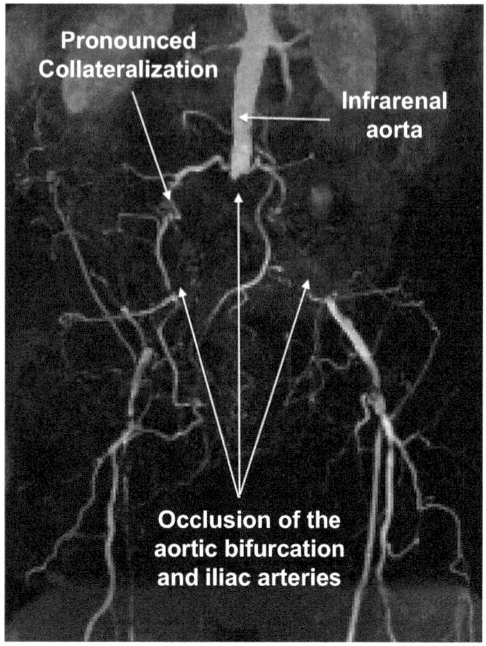

Fig. 40.1 Angiographic depiction of advanced multilevel peripheral arterial occlusive disease with chronic aortic occlusion (chronic Leriche syndrome) and pronounced collateralization

- Sometimes also abdominal and lumbar pain
- Shock symptoms are rather rare
- Not infrequently, "emergency" presentation by a general practitioner due to a sonographically or CT/MR angiographically diagnosed supposedly acute aortic occlusion, which is actually chronic and asymptomatic due to collateral circulation

Diagnostics

- Examination
  - pay attention to skin color, especially any cyanotic discoloration of the legs or of the buttocks and hips
  - assess pulse status
  - inguinal pulses are typically not palpable
  - determine ABI
  - often < 0.5
- Sonography
  - can be performed as an initial assessment if the device is available
  - otherwise, do not lose time and proceed with further diagnostics
- CT angiography
  - Assessment of the vessel wall
    - usually heavily calcified
    - sometimes visible stents

  - Assessment of the occlusion
    - calcified
    - fresh
    - "Bacon thrombus" may also appear fresh due to the low calcium content, but is often already older
- MRA
  - in principle possible, but takes longer and the vessel wall cannot be visualized as well
  - in addition, CT can also detect tumors or other abnormalities that are not visualized in MRA

Therapy
- Conservative
  - Indications:
    chronic or minimally symptomatic occlusion
    non-salvageable limb (Rutherford III)
    terminal/inoperable patient
  - Approach:
    antiplatelet therapy
    heparin infusion
    pain management (if necessary, morphine infusion)
- Interventional
  - Indications:
    depending on extent and length of occlusion, open or endovascular treatment
    in this regard, orientation according to TASC-II classification is possible
    A to D (A: short segment, mild; D: long segment, bilateral, with vessel branches such as the internal iliac artery or renal artery)
      A: endovascular
      B: preferably endovascular
      C: preferably open
      D: open
  - Approach:
    stent PTA
    CERAB procedure ("covered endovascular repair of aortic bifurcation")
- Surgical
  - Indications:
    In acute Leriche syndrome, there is an emergency indication, but with high risk of complications and time pressure.
    In acute but compensated symptoms, urgent early elective treatment (the next working day) can be performed.
    In compensated symptoms and chronic occlusion in TASC stages C and D, elective treatment can be performed.
  - Approach:
    transfemoral embolectomy and direct suture (in case of transverse arteriotomy) or

patch angioplasty in case of longitudinal arteriotomy and often additionally required thromboendarterectomy at the femoral bifurcation
if unsuccessful, then aortobiiliac or aortobifemoral reconstruction

Call the on-call service at night?

- In acute ischemia Rutherford IIb and/or compartment syndrome, emergency reconstruction and fasciotomy should be performed.
- In compensated ischemia Rutherford I or even IIa, it is usually possible to wait until the next morning.
- In Rutherford III ischemia and/or refusal of invasive therapy, it is also often possible to wait until the next morning.

Tips and Tricks

- If possible and justifiable, do not operate immediately as an emergency, but prepare and bowel prep the patient (e.g., overnight) beforehand.
- In some cases, surgery via the groin is possible, especially in arrhythmia and suspected embolism.
- If the presumed thrombus cannot be passed with a Fogarty catheter from the femoral approach, it may be a "fatty thrombus," and open reconstruction may be necessary.
- Shock symptoms are rather rare.
- Always consider ruptured aneurysm as a differential diagnosis.
- In patients with pre-existing PAD, the chances of success are lower, as a simple thrombectomy of the pelvic arteries is rarely feasible. Recanalization including stent implantation is often significantly more complex and the chances of success are lower.
- Generously prep and drape the patient up to the chest in a sterile fashion to allow for the possibility of creating an axillo(bi)femoral bypass if necessary.

Continuation of Case Study

The patient is clearly suffering from an acute and moderately or uncompensated arterial occlusion. She is in sinus rhythm, so from a differential diagnostic perspective, an arterial thrombosis in the setting of pre-existing PAD is most likely. A "simple" embolic occlusion is rather unlikely. In this case, as so often, CTA is the diagnostic modality of choice. It not only allows localization of the occlusion, but also assessment of the arterial wall morphology, the type and structure of the occlusion, and the abdominal organs. For example, advanced malignancies with associated malignant thrombophilia can be the underlying cause of an acute arterial occlusion.

Septic Erosive Bleeding of the Aorta

41

Septic erosion bleeding is a very serious complication following endovascular as well as open aortic procedures and is associated with high mortality. Often, these cases are referred for consultation from gastroenterology, with demonstration of a prosthetic-enteric fistula during esophagogastroscopy (Fig. 41.1).

Case Example
A 64-year-old patient, who underwent open repair of an infrarenal aortic aneurysm with a tube graft 5 months ago, is brought to the emergency department by paramedics with abdominal pain and after a collapse. He is hemodynamically stable but in a severely reduced general condition. The surgical scars are unremarkably healed, and CTA shows a contained rupture of the proximal anastomosis, compressing the left renal artery, which remains perfused. The right renal artery appears unremarkable. The concerned wife asks whether another operation is necessary. What is your response?

Definition
- Infection-related aortic bleeding following interventional or surgical vascular reconstruction

Typical Patient
- History of aortic surgical or interventional reconstruction
- Often known inflammatory disease of a thoracic, mediastinal, or abdominal organ (e.g., pancreatitis, colitis) and fistula formation to the prosthesis
- Current or previously documented wound healing disorders
- Diabetics and smokers (especially obese, but also very thin individuals) are particularly prone to wound healing disorders
- Recurrent gastrointestinal bleeding in the case of aortoduodenal fistula

S. Regus, *Vascular Surgical Emergencies*,
https://doi.org/10.1007/978-3-662-72646-4_41

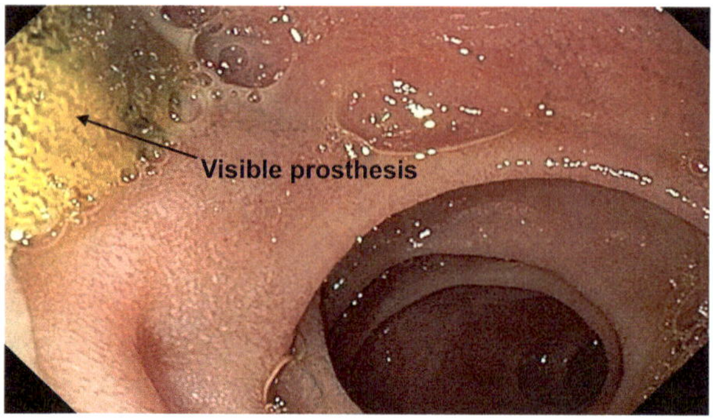

Fig. 41.1 Esophagogastroscopy reveals a large ulcer with visible portions of an aortic prosthesis in the setting of a fistula, melena, and infectious constellation. (Courtesy of Professor Pfister, Department of Vascular Surgery, University Hospital Regensburg)

- More common after aorto(bi)femoral reconstruction with bilateral groin incisions
- Less common after isolated laparotomy for aorto(bi)iliac reconstruction or isolated aortic procedures

Typical On-Call Scenario
- Often dramatically announced by emergency services as massive abdominal/inguinal/gastroduodenal bleeding in a patient with a known "aortic prosthesis"
- Usually via the emergency department/trauma bay
- Some patients also walk into the emergency department and report abdominal pain, fever, and abnormal discharge from their groin wounds/scars.
- Consultation requests from internal medicine (gastroenterology) or anesthesiology (intensive care unit) colleagues in case of abnormalities in gastroscopy or CT imaging

Diagnostics
- Clinical examination
  - of wounds/scars for redness, swelling, fluctuation
  - of peripheral circulation for pulses and sensorimotor function
- Swabs
  - initially obtain from open wounds (resistance testing takes time!)
- Laboratory
  - especially inflammatory markers
  - blood count
  - coagulation
- Ultrasound
  - can be very helpful in suspected abscess in the groin (anechoic formation)
  - however, in the case of abdominal infection, it is not always technically easy and often time-consuming

- CT angiography
  - diagnostic tool of choice
  - can be performed quickly
  - abscesses, bleeding sources, and infiltrations can be reliably visualized
  - air inclusions as an indication of infection
- PET-CT
  - for infection localization or
  - to rule out infection
- Aspiration
  - obtaining aspirate for bacteriological examination
  - indication for this must be very strict, as every aspiration carries the risk of bacterial contamination and thus infection
  - strict sterile precautions are essential and extremely important

Therapy

- Conservative
  - Indications:
    in stable condition
    without bleeding
    without sepsis
  - Procedure:
    Antibiotic therapy
    Pain management
    Follow-up monitoring (usually CTA)
- Interventional
  - Indications:
    in case of active bleeding
    hemorrhagic shock
    sepsis
  - Procedure:
    Aortic occlusion using a balloon for initial bleeding control = REBOA ("resuscitative endovascular balloon occlusion of the aorta")
    Implantation of a stent graft (aorta) or a covered stent (iliac or visceral vessels)
    Coil embolization of smaller branches
    as a permanent solution only possible if infection is ruled out
- Surgical
  - Indications:
    in case of massive bleeding
    after REBOA and stabilization of the patient
      →Important: Aortic occlusion should not be performed for more than 30 minutes!
    in case of clear infection of the prosthesis
    in case of rupture and endoleak

- Procedure:
  Explantation of the prosthesis
  Extra-anatomic reconstruction
  →axillo(bi)femoral
  →ideally before laparotomy, to keep the risk of bypass contamination as low as possible
  Anatomic reconstruction
  →prefer autologous replacement (e.g., with bovine pericardial patches from cardiac surgery)
  →alternatively, silver-coated prostheses

Call the on-call service at night?

- In the event of acute bleeding complications, hemodynamic instability, or septic clinical presentation, a telephone discussion of the procedure is necessary

Tips and Tricks

- Very serious clinical picture with high mortality
- Indicate antibiotic therapy liberally
- Broad-spectrum, anaerobes should be covered
- Piperacillin/tazobactam (e.g., Tazobac®) 4 g/0.5 g 1–1–1(–1)
- In case of penicillin allergy: meropenem (e.g., Meronem®) 1 g 1–1–1(–1)
- Indicate puncture in the groin or intra-abdominal/retroperitoneal region with extreme caution
- High risk of contamination!!
- Balloon occlusion (REBOA) can be used in emergencies in the shock room and is appropriate or even lifesaving, but occlusion should not last longer than 30 minutes

Case Study Continuation

This is a very critical clinical picture with high mortality, which is why you should definitely contact your on-call service. Until proven otherwise, in such a complication occurring several months after the initial procedure, infection must be assumed. Therefore, open reconstruction and explantation of the infected prosthesis as well as autologous or xenogeneic replacement would be indicated. In principle, endovascular management could also be considered as a bridging option; however, removal of all prosthetic components is necessary. An emergency surgical procedure for bleeding control is generally indicated.

42 Mesenteric Infarction

Mesenteric infarction (Fig. 42.1) is a clinical condition that is most often managed by colleagues in visceral surgery. Depending on the expertise available there, an intraoperative standby may be requested, or a consultative question may be posed regarding the indication for surgical or endovascular vascular reconstruction.

Case Example

An 82-year-old female patient is in the emergency department and is being treated by internal medicine. She reports abdominal pain that began about 12 hours ago and has now already improved. She has no history of abdominal surgery, is arrhythmic due to chronic atrial fibrillation, and also mentions having had diarrhea. The abdominal wall is tense and distended, but there are no signs of peritonism. Since the symptoms have significantly improved and the creatinine level is elevated at 3.1 mg/dl in the context of known renal insufficiency, the internal medicine colleague would like to admit the patient for observation and perform a CTA the following day. Do you agree with this approach?

Definition

- Occlusion of one (or more) of the three mesenteric arteries resulting in bowel ischemia:
  - Celiac trunk (TC)
  - Superior mesenteric artery (SMA)
  - Inferior mesenteric artery (IMA)
- The SMA is most commonly affected.
- TC and IMA are less commonly involved or rarely become symptomatic.

Typical Patient

- Older patient, women > men (approx. 4:1)
- Multimorbid

S. Regus, *Vascular Surgical Emergencies*,
https://doi.org/10.1007/978-3-662-72646-4_42

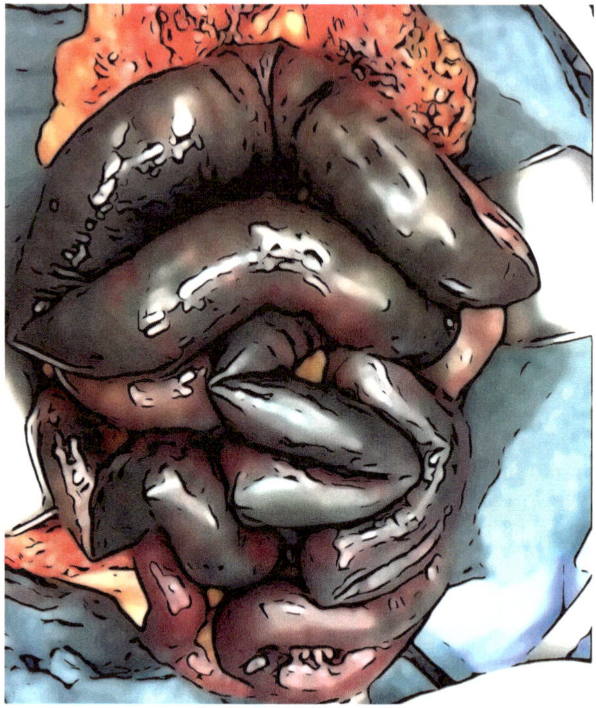

Fig. 42.1 Schematic illustration of irreversible mesenteric ischemia with "black" bowel

- Not infrequently with limited ability to communicate (dementia, from nursing home)
- Cardiac arrhythmias (most often chronic atrial fibrillation)

Typical On-Call Situation
- Often a consult from internal medicine or visceral surgery
- Abdominal pain with elevated lactate and assessment from a vascular surgery perspective requested
- Or assessment of CTA findings in the presence of mesenteric stenoses or occlusions in patients with abdominal pain
- Sometimes direct contact from visceral surgeons in the OR with an open abdomen and bowel ischemia

Diagnostics
- Examination
  - abdominal pain/acute abdomen
  - clinical findings can be misleading
    →Caution: "false peace" 6–12 h after onset of symptoms

- Laboratory tests (lactate, D-dimers, CK)
- Ultrasound
  - often non-diagnostic in the presence of meteorism!
- CT angiography
  - most important diagnostic tool
  - Assessment of visceral vessels
    SMA, IMA, or TC
    occlusion or stenoses
    extent of calcifications
  - Assessment of bowel wall
    air inclusions
    necroses
  - free air in the case of bowel gangrene and perforation

Therapy

- Conservative
  - Indications:
    if well compensated
    if inoperable
    if a generally present surgical indication is declined
    if the majority of the small intestine is "black" and incompatible with life
  - Approach:
    anticoagulation with heparin infusion
    antiplatelet therapy
    pain management
    → morphine infusion, if palliative situation
- Interventional
  - Indications:
    short-segment and calcified stenoses or occlusions
    in planned endovascular aortic stent procedures
  - Approach
    stent PTA (stand-alone PTA rarely promising)
- Surgical
  - Indications:
    in clear embolism and
    in suspected bowel ischemia
  - Approach:
    laparotomy
    if necessary, bowel resection and
    thrombectomy/embolectomy

Call the on-call service at night?

- Yes, because emergency reconstruction is indicated

Tips and Tricks

- TC and AMI are usually less important than the SMA, do not necessarily need to be reconstructed, and can be ligated if necessary.
- The SMA is most frequently affected by embolism and occlusive processes and is associated with clinical symptoms of ischemia.
- Not every occlusion of the visceral vessels discovered during further diagnostics is acute or causative for abdominal symptoms.
- If a laparotomy is planned and there are short-segment visceral occlusions, angiography with stent PTA should be performed beforehand. This offers the best chances for healing of intestinal anastomoses, and the resection margins during visceral surgery can be better assessed.
- In cases of extensive bowel wall damage (air inclusions = pneumatosis coli) and when, after opening the abdominal cavity, the entire bowel appears black, this finding is incompatible with life and palliative therapy is indicated.

Continuation of Case Example

Based on the described symptoms and examination findings, a mesenteric infarction must also be considered in the differential diagnosis. In this case, regression of symptoms is by no means reassuring, but could correspond to a "false peace." Waiting until the following day would be a death sentence for the patient, which is why, despite elevated renal values, an emergency CTA should be performed.

Ruptured Visceral Artery Aneurysm 43

The ruptured visceral artery aneurysm (Fig. 43.1) is also a rare aneurysm location, but one associated with a very high mortality rate. Under elective conditions, invasive exclusion carries an extremely low complication rate.

Case Example
A 46-year-old alcoholic with known alcohol-induced pancreatitis and multiple previous abdominal surgeries presents with an acute abdomen and hemorrhagic shock due to intra-abdominal bleeding. CT reveals a contained rupture of an aneurysm of the pancreaticoduodenal artery with an estimated diameter of 4 cm. There is great commotion and the patient is to be taken straight to the OR. Do you perhaps have another idea?

Definition
- Rupture of an aneurysm of a visceral artery
- Frequencies: splenic artery (60 %) > hepatic artery (30 %) > celiac trunk (5 %) > superior mesenteric artery (5 %)
- True aneurysm: most commonly splenic artery
- False aneurysm: often peripancreatic

Typical Patient
- True aneurysms:
  - often younger patients with a cardiovascular risk profile
  - women > men
- False aneurysms:
  - usually middle-aged patients with a history of alcohol use (alcohol-induced pancreatitis), obesity, and gallstones (biliary pancreatitis), or after laparoscopy (iatrogenic)
  - men > women

S. Regus, *Vascular Surgical Emergencies*,
https://doi.org/10.1007/978-3-662-72646-4_43

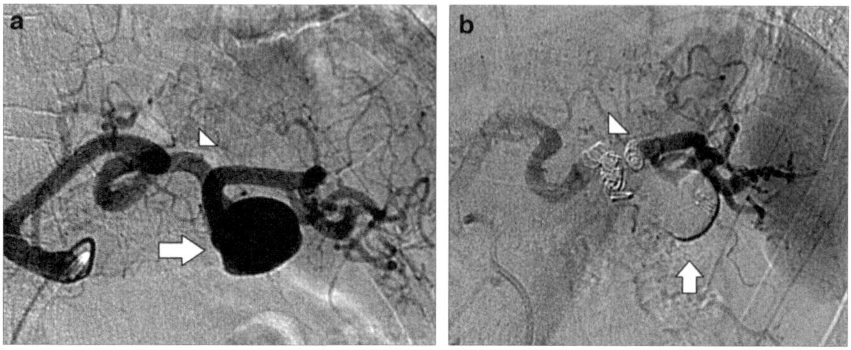

Fig. 43.1 a, b **a** Angiographic depiction of an aneurysm of the splenic artery before coil embolization (arrowhead: feeding artery, arrow: aneurysm sac), **b** Aneurysm of the splenic artery after successful coil embolization (arrowhead: coils in the afferent and efferent artery; arrow: aneurysm sac no longer perfused).

- Complains of recurrent abdominal pain, colicky or belt-like in nature
- Sometimes already known to have aortic, iliac, or popliteal aneurysms

Typical On-Call Situation
- Patient presents via emergency department, hemodynamically unstable, abdominal pain, suspected diagnosis of intra-abdominal bleeding of unclear origin
- Consult request from the ward (usually gastroenterology) for suspected visceral artery aneurysm (ultrasound) or abnormal CT finding
- Referral from visceral surgery after laparoscopy and now, on imaging, a visceral pseudoaneurysm (usually asymptomatic)
- Consult from gynecology regarding management of a visceral artery aneurysm in a pregnant woman (most often splenic artery)

Diagnostics
- Clinical examination
  - often asymptomatic
  - sometimes abdominal pain up to acute abdomen in case of rupture
  - pulsatile swelling palpable only in thin patients or with very large aneurysms
- Laboratory
  - anemia
  - elevated lactate in ileus/subileus
  - inflammatory markers in suspected pancreatitis
  - congestion parameters if cholangitis is suspected
  - liver and pancreatic enzymes in suspected alcohol abuse
- Ultrasound
  - abnormalities in pancreas/bowel/liver
  - visualization of the aneurysm (often difficult in the presence of meteorism)

- differentiation between true/false and size determination
- intra-/retroperitoneal bleeding
- CT angiography
  - confirmation of the diagnosis
  - size and diameter
  - true or false
  - active bleeding and extent of hematoma
  - abnormalities in bowel, liver, pancreas, spleen

Therapy

- Conservative
  - Indications:
    asymptomatic true aneurysm with diameter < 2 cm
    inoperability/refusal of invasive therapy
  - Approach:
    regular follow-up examinations
    treatment of risk factors:
    → smoking cessation
    → best medical treatment (BMT)
    → antihypertensive agents
    → antiplatelet therapy
    → statins
- Interventional
  - Indications:
    regardless of diameter
    → symptomatic/ruptured aneurysm
    → false aneurysm (unpredictable risk of rupture)
    → any aneurysm in women of childbearing age (increased risk of rupture during pregnancy)
    asymptomatic > 2 cm or increase in size > 0.5 cm/year
    anatomically feasible
  - Approach:
    covered stent
    coil embolization
    liquid embolization (with Onyx® = ethylene-vinyl alcohol copolymer)
- Surgical
  - Indications:
    same as interventional
    additionally, unsuccessful outcome after intervention and
    hemostasis including hematoma evacuation required
  - Approach:
    ligation if good backflow, otherwise interposition graft or bypass
    resection and end-to-end anastomosis (if kinking/elongation of the artery) or placement of an interposition graft (autologous)

Call the on-call service at night?

- In cases of emergency surgical indication with hemorrhagic shock, severe pain symptoms, or acute abdomen, support from visceral surgeons during laparotomy is desirable.

Tips and Tricks

- Splenic artery aneurysm is the most common visceral artery aneurysm encountered regularly in clinical practice
- In women of childbearing age, invasive exclusion is always indicated, regardless of diameter, because
  - the risk of rupture is unpredictable and increased during pregnancy
  - high mortality for mother and child
- False aneurysms are often associated with alcohol abuse, chronic inflammation (cholecystitis), or previous laparoscopic surgeries
- If technically and anatomically feasible, the endovascular-interventional approach should always be preferred
- In pseudoaneurysms, exclusion is the main goal (e.g., with coils); reconstruction is rarely possible or necessary

Case Study Continuation

Given the critical condition and multiple previous abdominal surgeries, open reconstruction certainly carries a very high mortality risk. If the necessary expertise and resources are available in-house, interventional therapy by embolization (usually with coils) would be the treatment of choice. With this minimally invasive approach, the patient's chances of survival would be significantly better than with open reconstruction.

Portal Vein Thrombosis

44

Portal vein thrombosis is usually diagnosed and treated primarily by gastroenterology, and if necessary, by visceral surgery. Vascular surgery is only very rarely consulted, which is why it is worth recalling the anatomy (Fig. 44.1) (it is easy to forget if you do not deal with it regularly).

Case Study
A 23-year-old man was brought directly to the OR via the trauma bay after a fight resulting in severe abdominal trauma. Intraoperatively, a rupture of the left hepatic lobe with diffuse bleeding was found, so the portal vein was compressed with a tourniquet to control bleeding during hepatic suturing and partial resection. After release, thrombosis of the left portal vein branch was observed, while the right branch was patent, and the proper hepatic artery was also free of thrombus. Would you recommend thrombectomy of the left portal vein branch?

Definition
- Acute or chronic thrombosis of the portal vein (PV)

Typical Patient
- Often has undergone multiple previous surgeries
  - Laparotomy/re-laparotomy leads to adhesions/strictures
  - Laparoscopy can cause outflow disturbances due to pneumoperitoneum
- Usually has known inflammatory or malignant diseases of the abdominal organs
  - Liver cirrhosis
  - Pancreatitis/pancreatic carcinoma
  - Hepatitis/hepatocellular carcinoma
  - Cholangiocarcinoma
  - Appendicitis/diverticulitis
  - Colon carcinoma
- Thrombophilia (often paraneoplastic)

S. Regus, *Vascular Surgical Emergencies*,
https://doi.org/10.1007/978-3-662-72646-4_44

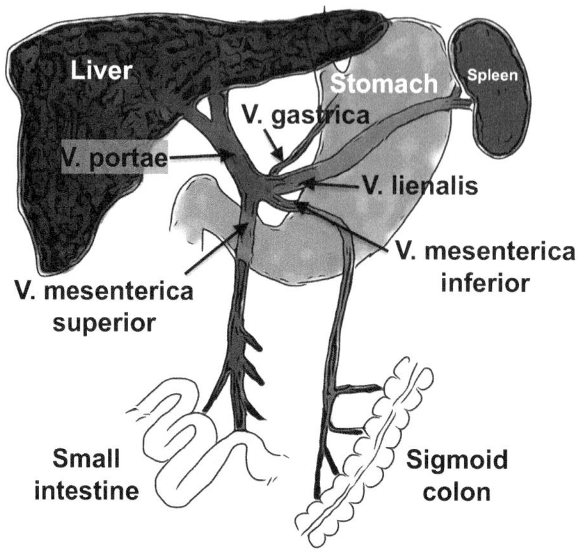

Fig. 44.1 Schematic representation of the portal vein and its tributaries

Typical On-Call Situation

- Usually a consult request from visceral surgery or gastroenterology
- Often an incidental finding of portal vein thrombosis on imaging
- Rarely, a call from the OR requesting assessment after laparotomy
- In "liver centers," as a complication after transplantation, possible indication for vascular surgery standby

Diagnostics

- Medical history
  - pre-existing inflammatory abdominal disease or liver cirrhosis
  - pancreatitis and alcohol abuse are a common combination
- Clinical examination
  - acute abdomen is rare
  - often relatively unremarkable examination findings
- Laboratory
  - coagulation parameters (liver function)
  - D-dimers (elevated in thrombosis)
  - liver function tests
- Ultrasound
  - often clearly visualized under good imaging conditions
  - difficult in cases of meteorism and obese abdominal wall
- CT
  - strongly recommended to confirm diagnosis
  - for planning invasive therapy

  - should always include **arterial** and **venous** phases
  - good visualization of the thrombosis and all surrounding structures
  - assessment of liver perfusion
  - assessment/extent of liver cirrhosis
- Gastroscopy
  - exclusion/detection of esophageal varices
- Rectoscopy
  - hemorrhoids (typical collateral circulation)

Therapy

- Conservative
  - Indications:
    asymptomatic patient
    short-segment thromboses with good collateral function
    inoperable patient
    poor overall prognosis
  - Approach:
    pain management
    therapeutic heparinization
    long-term anticoagulation with phenprocoumon or rivaroxaban
      →often spontaneous recanalization
      →but high risk of recurrence
- Interventional
  - Indications:
    confirmed acute thrombosis with pronounced portal venous congestion
    large or progressively enlarging esophageal varices
    liver failure
    impending mesenteric infarction
  - Approach:
    systemic thrombolytic therapy or
    local thrombolytic therapy via the superior mesenteric vein (retrograde principle)
    mechanical recanalization including stent implantation
      →usually as bridging or also
      →with palliative intent
    transjugular portosystemic shunt (TIPSS)
      →interventional procedure in which a shunt is created between the hepatic veins and the portal vein (usually the right branch) using a metal stent
- Surgical
  - Indications:
    unsuccessful interventional attempt
    bowel infarction
    liver failure
    progressive/rupture-prone esophageal varices

- Approach:
  thrombectomy
  portal vein replacement in case of tumor infiltration
  →partial resection and end-to-end anastomosis
  →placement of an interposition graft/bypass
  bowel resection in case of infarction
  liver transplantation

Call the on-call service at night?

- Rarely necessary, as the indication for emergency revascularization exists only in exceptional cases

Tips and Tricks

- Often chronic and an incidental finding with no need for intervention
- However, chronic consequences of portal vein thrombosis should not be underestimated (esophageal varices, rectal bleeding)
- Bowel infarctions are very rare and usually occur only with involvement of the mesenteric veins
- The Budd-Chiari syndrome should be known in this context:
  - outflow obstruction/thrombosis of the hepatic veins up to the inferior vena cava
  - etiology is diverse, usually a combination of thrombophilia and organ diseases (malignancies!)
- For complex or unclear findings, contact a “liver center” as early as possible

Continuation of Case Example

You would only need to perform a thrombectomy if both the portal vein (both branches) and the proper hepatic artery were occluded or transected. In the case described, however, only the left portal vein branch is occluded, which also supplies the injured and partially resected liver lobe. Therefore, a thrombectomy is not indicated and would even be contraindicated in this case. Keyword “damage control”: in such a polytraumatized patient, the surgical intervention should be as short as possible and focus on the most severe injuries that absolutely require treatment. The main goal is the survival of the patient (“getting them off the table alive”). After successful stabilization, further injuries and trauma consequences can still be managed as needed, but not in the emergency situation.

Thrombosis of the Mesenteric Veins 45

Thrombosis of the mesenteric veins (Fig. 45.1), like portal vein thrombosis, falls within the domain of gastroenterology and visceral surgery. This rare clinical picture can, with few exceptions, be managed conservatively and is often caused by malignant or inflammatory diseases of the intestine or liver.

Case Example
The on-call radiologist contacts you because he is currently reporting the CT scan of an internal medicine patient with acute pancreatitis of alcoholic etiology. He notes a short-segment thrombosis of the superior mesenteric vein; the portal vein and inferior mesenteric vein are free of thrombus, and the bowel appears unremarkable. In the meantime, the responsible colleagues from gastroenterology have also submitted a consultation request and are asking for a treatment recommendation. What do you write?

Definition
- Thrombosis of one or more mesenteric veins resulting in mesenteric infarction (infarct = arterial inflow problem, **infarction = venous** outflow problem)
- Affected veins:
  - Superior mesenteric vein
  - Inferior mesenteric vein
  - Portal vein

Typical Patient
- Unclear abdominal pain
- Symptoms present for several days (in contrast to arterial occlusion, which is acute)
- Current or previous history of inflammatory abdominal disease (pancreatitis, cholangitis, hepatitis, diverticulitis, colon cancer)

S. Regus, *Vascular Surgical Emergencies*,
https://doi.org/10.1007/978-3-662-72646-4_45

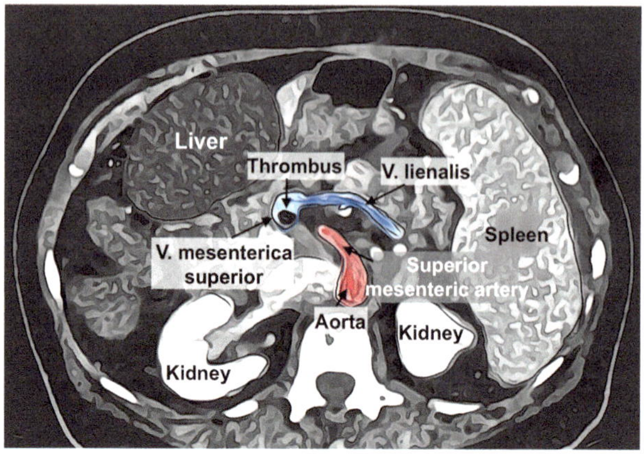

Fig. 45.1 Schematic representation of a thrombosis of the superior mesenteric vein at the confluence of the inferior mesenteric vein and the splenic vein

- Status post recent visceral surgery
- Status post blunt abdominal trauma (= posttraumatic)
- Thrombophilia (= paraneoplastic)

Typical On-Call Situation
- Usually initial evaluation and admission by internal medicine or visceral surgery
- Consultation request due to abdominal pain and CT-visible thrombosis

Diagnostics
- Clinical examination
  - usually unremarkable physical findings
  - mild to moderate abdominal tenderness
  - rarely guarding and "board-like" abdominal wall
  - suggests acute abdomen due to perforation/peritonitis
- Laboratory
  - Blood count (anemia, thrombocytosis, leukocytosis)
  - Coagulation
  - D-dimers
- ECG
  - usually unremarkable
  - no arrhythmias (as are often seen in arterial embolism)
- CT
  - with arterial and venous phase
- Phlebo-/angiography
  - only if intervention is planned

Therapy

- Conservative
  - Indications:
    mild pain symptoms
    exclusion of bowel ischemia or perforation
  - Approach:
    Heparin
      → preferably via syringe pump
      → successfully feasible in >70% of cases
      → very good spontaneous recanalization
      → alternatively, weight-adjusted LMWH
    Pain medication
      → paracetamol for mild pain
      → piritramide or morphine for more severe pain
    Antibiotics in case of infection
      → important here: efficacy against anaerobes
      Piperacillin/tazobactam (e.g., Tazobac®) 4 g/0.5 g 1–1–1(–1)
      in case of penicillin allergy, meropenem (e.g., Meronem®) 1 g 1–1–1(–1)
- Interventional
  - Indications:
    unsuccessful attempt at conservative therapy
    increasing pain symptoms
    (incipient) infarction
    if there is suspicion of a simultaneous arterial inflow problem
  - Approach:
    Phlebo-/angiography with readiness for intervention
    intravascular thrombolytic therapy
    if necessary, percutaneous transluminal angioplasty (PTA)/stent to rapidly improve perfusion and shorten the duration of laparotomy
- Surgical
  - Indications:
    bowel ischemia
    bowel gangrene
    suspected perforation
    "acute abdomen"
  - Approach:
    Indication for (exploratory) laparotomy should be set generously
    Thrombectomy
      → high risk of immediate re-occlusion with venous thrombectomy
      → arterial thrombectomy is essential, possibly with patch/bypass
    Bowel resection in case of gangrene
    "Second look" as determined by the surgeon

Call the on-call service at night?

- Rarely necessary, as patients are usually stable and the procedure is determined by visceral surgeons.
- However, if colleagues require a vascular surgeon during a visceral surgical procedure or announce this in advance, the on-call service should be informed.

Tips and Tricks

- The difference between infarction and infarzierung is mostly academic
  - Infarction results from an arterial inflow problem
  - Infarzierung is the result of a venous outflow problem
- It is usually only during surgery that it becomes clear whether the problem is arterial, venous, or combined
- The majority of isolated mesenteric vein thromboses can be successfully treated conservatively
- **Caution:** Time is critical in mesenteric infarction! Do not delay surgery for preoperative diagnostics in pursuit of precise knowledge of the etiology! Knowing whether the problem is arterial or venous does not change the approach. However, any delay before laparotomy can significantly worsen the patient's prognosis.

Continuation of Case Example

Even though it is often handled differently, one should not only assess the patient based on imaging but also clinically. The patient is in a very reduced state, cachectic, and has a distended, elastic abdominal wall without signs of peritonism. There is no indication for operative or interventional recanalization; depending on comorbidities, however, therapeutic administration of heparin may be considered. The main focus should certainly be on treating the pancreatitis with fasting and infusion therapy, and, if necessary, further evaluation and tumor search.

Part XI
Complications

Postoperative Carotid Occlusion

46

Postoperative carotid occlusion (Fig. 46.1), a fortunately rare complication of carotid surgery, occurs in the majority of cases within the first few hours postoperatively, sometimes even still in the operating room. In the vast majority of cases, technical errors are the cause, most often anastomotic stenoses or embolizations during preparation or after release of the anastomosis.

Case Example
A 68-year-old patient underwent right-sided carotid reconstruction with an unremarkable intraoperative course. You were the first assistant and performed the skin closure while the operating senior physician had already left and was completing the surgical documentation. After extubation, weakness of the left arm and, to a lesser extent, the left leg is noted. The senior physician cannot be reached by phone, and the anesthesiologist asks you whether he should take the patient directly to the CT scan. What do you do?

Definition

- Occlusion of the carotid arteries, usually the internal carotid artery (ICA), less commonly the external carotid artery (ECA) or common carotid artery (CCA)
- Directly following surgical reconstruction

Typical Patient

- Patient immediately after surgical carotid reconstruction
- More common in symptomatic than in asymptomatic stenoses
- Women, diabetics, and recurrent stenoses are also more frequently affected

Typical On-Call Situation

- Neurologically abnormal patient in the recovery room, intensive care unit, or general ward

S. Regus, *Vascular Surgical Emergencies*,
https://doi.org/10.1007/978-3-662-72646-4_46

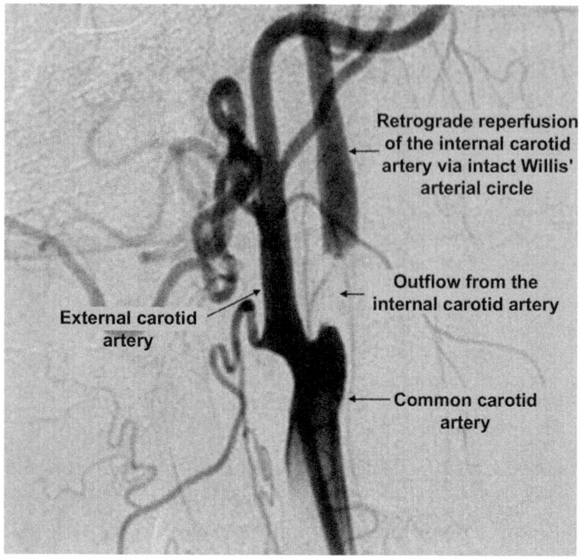

Fig. 46.1 Angiographic depiction of an acute postoperative occlusion of the internal carotid artery (ICA) after eversion endarterectomy

- Sometimes already directly during the operation (regional anesthesia) or after extubation (general anesthesia with neuromonitoring and/or shunt) neurological abnormalities in the sense of ipsilateral ischemia in the middle cerebral artery territory

Diagnostics
- Clinical examination
  - if still in the operating room, this is sufficient
  - no further diagnostics, proceed directly to exploration
- Sonography
  - for orientation only
  - cross-sectional imaging indicated to confirm diagnosis
- CCT and CTA
  - if symptoms occur outside the operating room
  - urgently and without significant delay: Time is brain!

Therapy
- Conservative
  - Indications:
    if CTA excludes both extra- and intracranial carotid occlusion and
    no embolism is visible
    no infarction, but hemorrhage (directly postoperatively often due to hypertensive crises)

if massive infarction and findings are incompatible with life (presumed patient wishes are decisive)
  - Approach:
    Monitoring in the stroke unit
    CCT follow-up scans
    strict blood pressure monitoring (hypo- and hypertensive crises must be prevented)
- Interventional
  - Indications:
    in isolated dissection in the operative area
    in case of embolization to the intracranial vessels
    if surgery was performed some time ago and there is significant scarring
    at the patient's request
  - Approach:
    Stent implantation is generally possible, but surgical revision should be preferred
    if necessary, aspiration thrombectomy
    thrombolysis is contraindicated
- Surgical
  - Indications:
    almost always indicated and should be preferred
  - Approach:
    Revision of the anastomosis and, if necessary, central thrombectomy (with Fogarty catheter)
    Hematoma evacuation

Call the on-call senior physician at night?
- No compromises: Always call in case of complications after carotid procedures!

Tips and Tricks
- In case of abnormalities immediately postoperatively (still in the operating room), do not initiate further diagnostics, but immediately explore the wound and check the anastomosis.
- During surgical revision, placement of an interposition graft is often necessary. For this, alloplastic material is usually used; the ECA can and is often ligated and divided due to better anastomotic geometry.

Continuation of Case Study
Since the intraoperative course was uneventful, it is highly likely that a technical problem has occurred; presumably, the thrombendarterectomized carotid artery has acutely occluded. CT imaging is not indicated, as it would only result in unnecessary loss of time. You ask the anesthesiologist to keep the patient in the operating room, to induce anesthesia, and the surgical staff to prepare everything for an immediate revision procedure.

Bypass Occlusion

47

Bypass occlusion is an acute emergency that must be promptly treated in the acute ischemia stage according to Rutherford IIb. Otherwise, with prolonged and ultimately irreversible ischemia, there is a risk of limb loss (Fig. 47.1).

Case Study

A 62-year-old female smoker is referred by her general practitioner, who suspects a recurrent occlusion of her femoropopliteal bypass. She reports exertional pain with a reduction in walking distance to 50 m. Previously, she was able to walk several kilometers without difficulty. Placement of a synthetic bypass below the knee joint (=FP-III-PTFE) was performed at another hospital 2 years ago, also due to exertional calf pain. On examination, the affected foot is warm, sensorimotor function is completely intact, the ABI is 0.6, sonography shows the bypass is occluded, and the popliteal artery is monophasic. Do you order a CTA and arrange for invasive revascularization?

Definition

- Occlusion of a vascular graft or implant
- Acute or chronic

Typical Patient

- Often these are "old acquaintances" who return repeatedly.
- Typical "vascular patient" with a cardiovascular risk profile and history of multiple vascular interventions/reconstructions

Typical Situation on Duty

- Patients often present to the hospital/emergency department already diagnosed with a bypass occlusion, as they are very familiar with the symptoms.
- Sometimes, however, it is the first occlusion event or
- Immediate occlusion after surgery during the same hospital stay

S. Regus, *Vascular Surgical Emergencies*,
https://doi.org/10.1007/978-3-662-72646-4_47

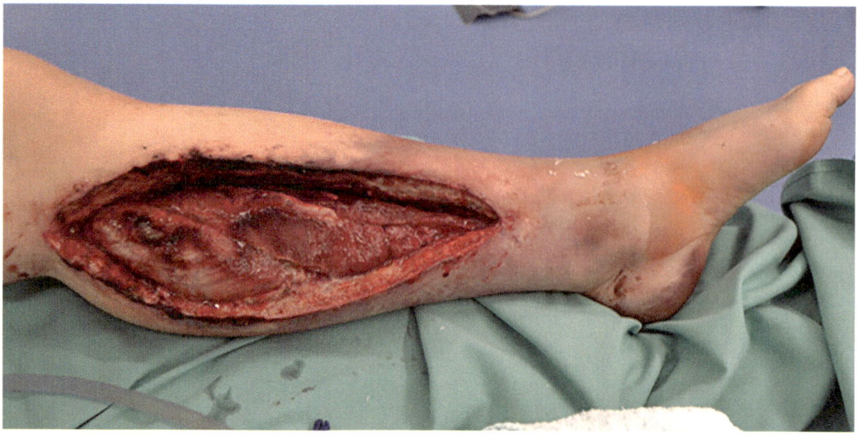

Fig. 47.1 Irreversible ischemia of the left lower leg due to prolonged ischemia and status post bypass revision with fasciotomy. Typical findings are nonviable necrotic wound edges and clay-like altered musculature

Diagnostics

- Clinical examination
  - cooler foot compared to the other side
  - possibly livid discoloration
  - reduced/absent sensorimotor function
  - Inspect surgical wounds/scars:
    anastomotic aneurysm?
    infection?
    hematoma?
    seroma?
    dehiscence?
    prosthesis visible?
- Doppler pressure measurement
  - usually ABI < 0.3 or not measurable
- Sonography
  - if findings are clear, further therapy can be indicated
- CT angiography
  - for therapy planning in unclear cases or
  - in central occlusions

Therapy

- Conservative
  - Indications:
    if asymptomatic (rare), then discuss conservative management
    in cases of mild symptoms (Rutherford I)
    in Rutherford III and refusal of amputation

- Approach:
  initially heparin as a bolus, usually 5000 IU
  then via perfusor, PTT 60–80
  palliative pain management with morphine perfusor
  →1–2 mg/h via perfusor (1 mg/ ml, infusion rate 1–2 ml/h)
- Interventional
  - Indications:
    in cases of mild symptoms (Rutherford I and IIa) with elective therapy planning
  - Approach:
    lysis or
    aspiration thrombectomy
- Surgical
  - Indications:
    in cases of moderately compensated symptoms (Rutherford IIa/b)
    in decompensated/irreversible ischemia (Rutherford III)
  - Approach:
    Thrombectomy
    Bypass creation
    Fasciotomy
    Amputation in irreversible ischemia
    →otherwise risk of death from systemic reperfusion syndrome

Call the on-call service at night?

- In a compensated situation, it is possible to wait until the next morning and treat the patient on the ward with a heparin perfusor.
- Thrombolysis can be initiated independently after consulting radiology, but it is best not to start this in the middle of the night. The risk of complications is significantly increased and rarely justified.
- In cases of critical ischemia (Rutherford IIb), bleeding complications, or suspected compartment syndrome, emergency revision is indicated and the on-call service must be contacted without fail.

Tips and Tricks

- Not every bypass occlusion detected on imaging (e.g., in CTA performed for other reasons) is acute and requires treatment.
- A typical scenario is, for example, a centralized patient with acute myocardial infarction after successful resuscitation and now with cool extremities due to occlusion of a femoropopliteal bypass seen on CTA. Not infrequently, intraoperatively or during intervention, this proves to be impassable and chronically occluded. In such cases, a conservative approach is recommended initially. After cardiac recompensation, peripheral perfusion often improves and returns to the baseline status (prior to cardiovascular failure and resuscitation).
- Always have a low threshold for performing fasciotomy in any surgical vascular reconstruction.

Continuation of Case Example

In the case of an infragenual femoropopliteal synthetic bypass and acute ischemia at Rutherford stage I, as well as a painless walking distance of 50 m, conservative therapy would be the treatment of choice. Therefore, a CT angiography would have no consequence, and both radiation and contrast agent exposure should be avoided. Invasive therapy would carry the risk of complications with worsening of symptoms, which would only be indicated in advanced stages of ischemia (Rutherford IIa or b). Many patients experience significant symptom improvement after the acute phase and can achieve a better outcome through structured walking training than through repeated bypass revisions. With each new bypass occlusion and subsequent revision, the risk of complications increases, which can ultimately lead to limb loss.

Bypass Infection

48

Infection of a bypass (Fig. 48.1) is limited to alloplastic implants and often requires explantation with autologous and/or extra-anatomic reconstruction.

Case Study
A "regular patient" is in the emergency department. Multiple vascular surgical procedures and revisions, most recently a surgical revision of the proximal anastomosis of a left supragenual femoropopliteal vein bypass using a bovine patch four weeks ago, are in his history. He now presents with swelling and redness in the left groin. The surgical scar is dehiscent, there is putrid secretion, and the bypass tract on the thigh appears clinically as a reddened cord. You want to know if the bypass is patent, which can already be confirmed clinically by palpable foot pulses and a warm foot. CT shows a localized collection with air inclusions in the groin; the bypass is perfused and on the thigh without surrounding fluid rim. What do you do?

Definition
- Infection of an implant by pathogens
- Usually develops locally, rarely systemic septic dissemination

Typical Patient
- Patient after bypass placement
- Almost exclusively alloplastic implants
- Recent bypass placement with wound healing disorders
- Longer-standing cases with known aneurysms (mostly groin)
- Diabetics and smokers at risk, as well as obese and very thin patients

Typical On-Call Situation
- Patient shortly after bypass placement on the ward now with abnormal wounds, putrid secretion, fever, or

S. Regus, *Vascular Surgical Emergencies*,
https://doi.org/10.1007/978-3-662-72646-4_48

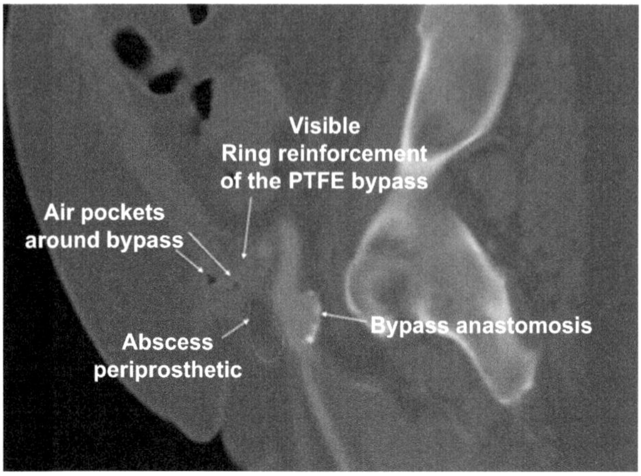

Fig. 48.1 CTA of an infected crossover bypass with air inclusions and abscess formation around the bypass

- Referral from a general practitioner after bypass placement and the above findings
- Presentation to the emergency department with increasing pain in the area of the surgical wounds or scars
- Hemorrhagic shock due to bleeding in the anastomosis area of a bypass (mostly groin)

Diagnostics
- Clinical examination
  - already externally visible redness along the bypass
  - redness and dehiscence in the wound area
  - pulsatile swelling in case of anastomotic aneurysm
  - often a combination of infection with occlusion, so also watch for signs of ischemia
- Laboratory
  - inflammatory markers (leukocytes, CRP, procalcitonin PCT)
- Bacteriological examinations
  - swab
- Ultrasound
  - hypoechoic or anechoic rim around the bypass in combination with signs of infection is highly suggestive of a bypass infection
- CT angiography
  - diagnostic tool of choice
  - findings suggestive of infection: abscesses, air inclusions, contrast-enhancing formations around the bypass
  - bypass occlusion visible
  - erosive bleeding visible
  - if diagnosis remains unclear, possibly PET-CT (positron emission tomography-CT)

Therapy

- Conservative
  - Indications:
    externally unremarkable findings and
    no systemic signs of infection
    no or well-compensated occlusion
    preferably in autologous bypasses
  - Procedure:
    Antibiotic therapy, usually i.v. with broad spectrum, e.g., piperacillin/tazobactam (e.g., Tazobac®) 4 g/0.5 g 4×daily
    Cooling
    Pain management
- Interventional
  - Indications:
    bypass occlusion moderately compensated (Rutherford I and IIa)
    locally limited abscess formation
    retroperitoneal abscess formation in close proximity to aorto- or iliacofemoral reconstructions
    inoperable patient with erosion bleeding
  - Procedure:
    Bypass lysis, e.g., with Actilyse®
    Abscess puncture and bacteriological examination
    Percutaneous placement of a suction/irrigation drain
    Implantation of a coated stent/stent graft in case of bleeding as a bridging measure
- Surgical
  - Indications:
    massive bleeding in the anastomosis area
    bypass infected along its entire length with systemic signs of infection
    decompensated or irreversible ischemia
  - Procedure:
    Bypass explantation with application of a VAC dressing
    anatomic reconstruction, if autologous/xenogeneic is possible
    extra-anatomic reconstruction, e.g., axillofemoral or obturator bypass, if only alloplastic is possible
    major amputation in case of irreversible ischemia

Call the on-call service at night?

- In most cases, it is sufficient to admit the patient to the hospital, administer antibiotics, and report during the morning round. Emergency surgery is rarely indicated.
- In cases of erosion bleeding, septic clinical picture, or critical ischemia with bypass occlusion (Rutherford IIb), the on-call service should be informed.

Tips and Tricks

- Do not puncture an unremarkable seroma, as this may lead to contamination with pathogens
- An anechoic rim around a synthetic bypass may represent a sterile "perigraft reaction." Here too: Do not puncture if there are no external signs of irritation and no local or systemic signs of infection
- Conspicuous wound/scar conditions should never be spread under non-sterile conditions on the ward, but always in the OR and under sterile precautions

Continuation of Case Example

You indicate operative groin revision and prescribe an antibiotic. The procedure must be performed under strict sterile conditions and under general anesthesia. The leg should be completely prepped, ideally also the contralateral leg, in order to possibly harvest the great saphenous vein. If only an abscess is found, it may be drained and initially treated with open wound management. In the vast majority of cases, however, explantation of the bypass and autogenous reconstruction are necessary.

Postoperative Rebleeding

49

Severe postoperative bleeding complications (Fig. 49.1) from one's own cases, as well as intraoperative bleeding that is difficult to control in other specialties, are the business of vascular surgery. One should always, and especially "without complaint," offer assistance, even if no vascular surgery "standby" was previously requested.

Case Example

You are called to see a 78-year-old multimorbid female patient who underwent a femoral bifurcation thromboendarterectomy with patch angioplasty earlier today. She is hemodynamically unstable, with a systolic blood pressure of 100 mmHg and a heart rate of 120/min. The Redon drain is full, and the operated groin shows a large hematoma with tense soft tissue swelling. The responsible nurse reports a hemoglobin value of 6.2 g/dl and asks whether the patient needs a CTA. What is your response?

Definition

- Bleeding/rebleeding is a common complication after surgical procedures, especially in vascular surgery.
- A distinction is made between diffuse bleeding (often manageable conservatively) and anastomotic insufficiency (requiring revision).

Typical Patient

- Often elderly patients with pre-existing anticoagulation
- Repeat interventions
- Complex reconstructions
- Central > peripheral procedures

S. Regus, *Vascular Surgical Emergencies*,
https://doi.org/10.1007/978-3-662-72646-4_49

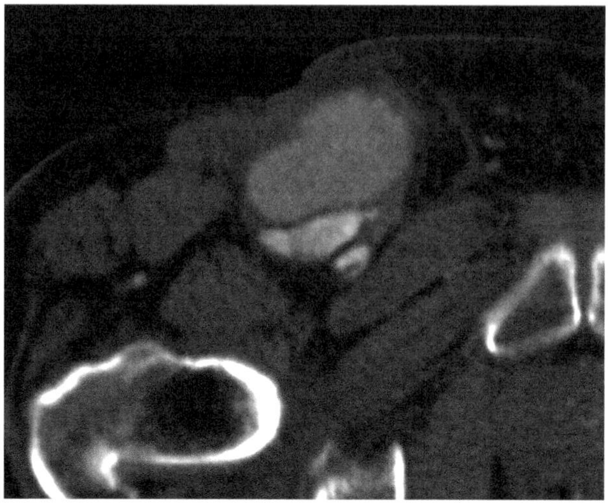

Fig. 49.1 Postoperative rebleeding after femoral patch angioplasty and subsequent emergency surgical revision and hemostasis

Typical On-Call Situation

- Hematoma in the surgical area, pain, possibly circulatory problems
- Dysphagia, possibly dyspnea after carotid procedures
- For central procedures, often presents as an emergency on the ward or intensive care unit with hemodynamic instability as an indication of significant bleeding
- Blood-soaked dressing after toe amputation
- Groin hematoma after femoral thromboendarterectomy

Diagnostics

- Clinical findings
  - are usually decisive
  - visible hematoma
  - bleeding from the surgical wound
  - pulsatile swelling
  - hemodynamic instability
  - Caution: Do not lose time with further diagnostics if the patient is unstable!
- Laboratory tests (blood count, coagulation)
- Ultrasound
  - extent of the hematoma
  - active bleeding
- CT angiography
  - diagnostic tool of choice if the patient is stable and a central procedure was performed
  - no delay if there is clear evidence of bleeding complication and hemodynamic instability

Therapy

- Conservative
  - Indications:
    for diffuse bleeding due to coagulopathy and
    exclusion of anastomotic insufficiency
    no hemodynamic relevance
  - Approach:
    pause anticoagulation
    if necessary, administer protamine or PCC
    compression (sandbag to groin)
- Interventional
  - Indications:
    bleeding from a side branch or dissection/perforation after percutaneous transluminal angioplasty (PTA)
    intracerebral bleeding after carotid procedure
  - Approach:
    placement of a covered stent
    embolization with coils/alcohol
- Surgical
  - Indications:
    postoperative patient is unstable with increasing hematoma in the surgical area
    clear anastomotic insufficiency
    cervical bleeding with progressive dyspnea/dysphagia
  - Approach:
    take the patient back to the OR and control the bleeding
    if necessary, optimize coagulation beforehand
    have packed red blood cells available

Call the on-call service at night?

- When in doubt, always make contact, especially in cases of
  - complications from surgery performed the same day
  - active bleeding
  - large, tense hematoma
  - tension blisters
  - increasing pain
  - suspected anastomotic tear or
  - impending bypass occlusion
  - cervical hematoma increasing in size with signs of compression

Tips and Tricks

- Be cautious after central procedures and carotid surgery: life-threatening complications can occur here, so be liberal and early in indicating surgery
- An unstable patient, especially after a central procedure, should be taken to the OR immediately

- In cases of cervical rebleeding, it may be necessary in emergencies (non-sterile) to remove the suture material and decompress the hematoma so that the anesthesiologist can intubate
- Decompress cervical hematoma after carotid intervention liberally and early, as otherwise severe complications can develop on the regular ward
- A groin hematoma can sometimes be successfully compressed
- Even larger hematomas in the extremities can sometimes be managed conservatively (compression, sandbag, coagulation optimization). However, monitor closely: even if the bleeding stops, compression can result in bypass occlusion
- Rebleeding after toe amputation can often be compressed; sometimes ligation and coagulation are necessary and effective
- If possible, at the end of vascular surgery (after restoration of blood flow), heparin should be antagonized with protamine
- In cases of rebleeding, always check and, if necessary, optimize coagulation

Continuation of Case Example

You inform the nurse that the patient must be taken to the OR as an emergency, without detour via CT, and together you apply a compression bandage. The diagnosis of rebleeding is clear, and every minute of delay worsens the patient's prognosis. You inform the on-call service, the anesthesia colleagues, and the OR nursing staff about the emergency indication.

50 Ischemic Colitis After Aortic Procedures

In ischemic colitis (Fig. 50.1), the key principle is: thinking of it is most important. Especially after an initially unremarkable postoperative course following open aortic surgery, if there is clinical deterioration with increasing abdominal pain between the 3rd and 6th postoperative day, further diagnostic workup (CTA and rectoscopy) should be initiated.

Case Example

An 83-year-old patient with an initially uncomplicated course after aortobifemoral Y-graft placement for bilateral common iliac artery aneurysms and an abdominal aortic aneurysm is already on the regular ward and, although his diet was advanced somewhat slowly, he ultimately tolerated it without problems. Now, however, he complains of increasing abdominal pain, and the nurse reports that he has a fever (38.9°C). He has tenderness in the left lower abdomen and appears very frail. Laboratory tests show elevated inflammatory markers, but hemoglobin and erythrocytes are within the normal range. What is your suspicion?

Definition

- Postoperative colonic ischemia after open or endovascular aortic procedures

Typical Patient

- Patient with an infrarenal aortic aneurysm and recent surgical repair within the last few days
- Usually with additional stenoses of the visceral arteries (most commonly the superior mesenteric artery [SMA]) or iliac arteries (internal iliac artery [IIA])
- Typical cardiovascular risk profile, with tobacco abuse being most prominent
- Intraoperative ligation or overstenting of the iliac arteries

S. Regus, *Vascular Surgical Emergencies*,
https://doi.org/10.1007/978-3-662-72646-4_50

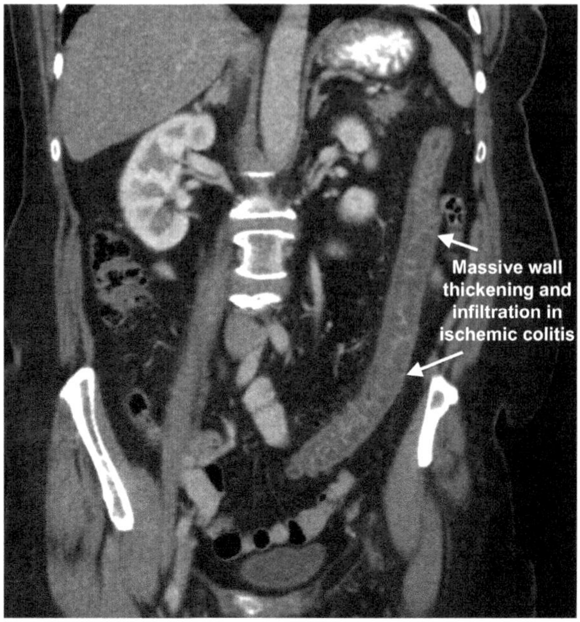

Fig. 50.1 In a patient with ischemic colitis of the descending colon and sigmoid, CT shows massive wall thickening and infiltration

Typical On-Call Scenario

- Increasing abdominal pain after aortic surgery
  - typically on postoperative days 3–5
  - localized in the left mid/lower abdomen
- Clinical deterioration after an initially unremarkable immediate postoperative course
- Fever, (bloody) diarrhea, and rising inflammatory markers on postoperative days 2–3

Diagnostics

- Clinical examination
  - Patient often appears severely debilitated
  - Tenderness in the left lower/mid abdomen
  - Signs of peritonism
- Laboratory tests
  - Leukocytosis, sometimes leukopenia, elevated inflammatory markers (CRP, PCT)
  - Thrombocytopenia, decreased prothrombin time (Quick)
- Blood cultures
  - if fever and/or chills are present

- Ultrasound
  - thickened bowel wall
  - but often of limited value in the presence of meteorism
- CT angiography
  - rapid and reliable assessment of bowel and vessels
  - position of the graft and patency visible
  - thickened bowel wall can be visualized, possibly with intramural air
  - perfusion disturbance visible
  - free air in case of perforation
- Rectoscopy
  - ischemic mucosa visible
  - useful for diagnostic confirmation

Therapy
- Conservative
  - Indications:
    in cases of minor changes
    regression of symptoms
    exclusion of sepsis
    exclusion of (impending) bowel wall perforation
  - Procedure:
    i.v. antibiotics
      broad-spectrum including anaerobic coverage
      Piperacillin/Tazobactam (e.g., Tazobac®) 4 g/0.5 g 1–1–1(–1)
      Meropenem (e.g., Meronem®) 1 g 1–1–1(–1)
    heparin perfusor
    pain management
    nil by mouth and infusion therapy
    if necessary, Prostaglandin® 2 × 40 μg
- Interventional
  - Indications:
    in cases of stenosis of the visceral or iliac arteries
    in cases of thrombotic occlusions
  - Procedure:
    percutaneous transluminal angioplasty (PTA)
    often with stent
    local lysis therapy
    aspiration thrombectomy
- Surgical
  - Indications:
    prosthesis or limb occlusion
    prosthesis infection
    multisegmental occlusions
    bowel wall perforation (impending or manifest)

- Procedure:
  revision procedure from femoral approach if "only" limb occlusion
  re-laparotomy in case of prosthesis occlusion or infection
  if necessary, open surgical thrombectomy or embolectomy
  bowel resection

Call the on-call service at night?

- Bowel perforation or prosthesis occlusion are emergency indications, so contacting the on-call service is essential in these cases
- If the findings are stable after exclusion of (impending) perforation, it is sufficient to pass on the information the following day, provided the patient is nil by mouth, receiving antibiotics, and undergoing infusion therapy

Tips and Tricks

- Remembering this is essential and can be life-saving!
- A typical feature is deterioration of the clinical condition on the 2nd–3rd postoperative day after an initially unremarkable course
- Warning signs are fever, rising inflammatory markers, and peritonism
- Because the symptoms worsen insidiously, delayed diagnosis is not uncommon and bowel perforation is often already present. In such cases, patients have a high mortality rate, especially with fecal peritonitis and exposed prosthesis

Case Study Continuation

You should consider ischemic colitis, especially due to the left-sided abdominal pain, elevated inflammatory parameters, and the aortobiiac reconstruction with end-to-end anastomosis proximally and distally. With poor collateral function, perfusion disorders typically occur in the sigmoid and rectum. Performing a CTA is strongly recommended, as well as nil by mouth, administration of heparin, infusion therapy, and i.v. antibiotics. In case of suspected bowel perforation, re-laparotomy would be indicated.

51 Burst Abdomen

In particular, obese patients with lung diseases, chronic cough, as well as those who have undergone treatment for a ruptured aortic aneurysm with a large hematoma, are at increased risk for developing abdominal wound dehiscence (Fig. 51.1). A typical sign is persistent (meat broth-colored) secretion from the abdominal wound.

Case Example
In the intensive care unit, there is a patient who received an aortobifemoral Y-graft for PAD two days ago. He is obese, has known chronic obstructive pulmonary disease (COPD), and the nursing staff mentions that the abdominal dressings need to be changed constantly due to heavy secretion. You examine the dressing; the absorbent pads are soaked with clear yellow-brown fluid, and when pressure is applied, this secretion drains from the lower wound margin. How can you diagnose abdominal wound dehiscence?

Definition

- Insufficiency of fascial closure after laparotomy

Typical Patient

- Patient on a general or intensive care unit after open aortic surgery and transperitoneal approach (laparotomy) within hours to a few days
- Dressings typically need to be changed frequently by nursing staff due to increased secretion from the abdominal wound.
- On gentle pressure, clear fluid drains, often described as "meat broth-colored" secretion. This is peritoneal fluid.
- In some cases, small intestine may protrude from the wound if there is subcutaneous or cutaneous dehiscence.

S. Regus, *Vascular Surgical Emergencies*,
https://doi.org/10.1007/978-3-662-72646-4_51

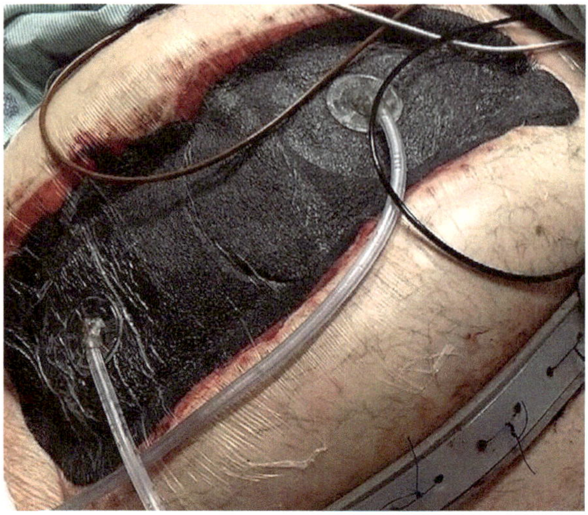

Fig. 51.1 Clinical finding in massive abdominal wound dehiscence managed with a VAC® dressing

- Risk factors include:
  - ruptured aneurysm with large hematoma, which cannot be fully decompressed in cases of diffuse tissue bleeding
  - nicotine abuse
  - chronic lung diseases, as these typically lead to intra-abdominal pressure spikes, e.g., during coughing fits
  - obesity

Typical On-Call Situation

- Usually, nursing staff on the ward contact you due to problems with wound care
- Less commonly, patients re-present via the emergency department due to wound dehiscence and increasing secretion after a recent (<14 days) transperitoneal vascular procedure with staples still in place
- If the surgery was performed longer ago, abdominal wound dehiscence is unlikely, and scar infections or hernias are more common.

Diagnostics

- Clinical examination
  - typical secretion of clear fluid (resembling meat broth)
  - wound dehiscence, usually below the umbilicus
  - possibly visible bowel wall
- Ultrasound
  - with standard B-mode, the fascia can usually be well assessed

- X-ray
  - if indicated, in two planes in suspected ileus or free air
  - in such cases, however, it is better to proceed directly to CT to save time
- CT
  - rarely necessary
  - in most cases, history, clinical findings, and ultrasound are sufficient to indicate surgical exploration
  - important in suspected ischemic colitis
  - the sigmoid and rectum are most commonly affected after ligation of the inferior mesenteric artery during aortic surgery
  - concurrent iliac stenosis/occlusion is an additional warning sign
  - most often manifests on postoperative days 3–6, rarely later

Therapy

- Conservative
  - Indications:
    in case of a small fascial defect and sufficient suture
    inoperability (e.g., terminal patient)
    in fecal peritonitis due to perforation with prolonged sigmoid ischemia as well as definitely contaminated/infected aortic prosthesis
    →usually a palliative situation
  - Procedure:
    Antibiotic therapy, e.g., piperacillin/tazobactam
    Protein substitution
    Wound care with highly absorbent materials
    if necessary, application of a VAC dressing
    possibly cutaneous revision with new suture/stapling
- Surgical
  - Indications:
    manifest burst abdomen
    intra-abdominal complications such as
      →bleeding
      →rebleeding
      →prosthesis infection
      →prosthesis occlusion
      →anastomotic insufficiency
      →ileus
      →hollow organ perforation
  - Procedure:
    Exploration
    if necessary, new fascial suture in case of partial insufficiency
    temporary abdominal wall closure with VAC dressing and "shoelace suture"
    elimination of intra-abdominal complications; for this, however, consult colleagues from visceral surgery at an early stage

Call the on-call service at night?

- A burst abdomen itself does not constitute an emergency indication, so if the patient is stable and intra-abdominal bleeding, infection, or hollow organ perforation are excluded, it is possible to wait until the next morning.
- Otherwise, in the case of the above-mentioned intra-abdominal complications, immediate emergency contact must be made.

Tips and Tricks

- Heavy secretion of clear, serosanguinous fluid shortly after laparotomy is usually due to burst abdomen
- Examine the infraumbilical abdominal wall closure particularly carefully, as fascial closure insufficiency most commonly occurs here
- In case of doubt, always explore in the operating room and prefer temporary abdominal wall closure
- Always look for and (ideally) treat the cause of burst abdomen preoperatively to avoid intraoperative surprises. The most common causes are:
  - coughing fits in COPD
  - ileus/subileus
  - ischemic colitis
  - bowel perforation (iatrogenic or ischemic)
- Request visceral surgical support early

Continuation of Case Example

You can either visualize the fascial defect sonographically, which is not always easy. You can also try to explore the wound dehiscence with sterile gloves and forceps. If you can palpate a fascial gap or penetrate very deeply with the forceps, then the diagnosis of burst abdomen is almost certain and surgical revision should be performed promptly. This does not necessarily have to take place in the middle of the night, but should be done promptly the following day—preferably not at the end of the regular OR schedule.

Compartment Syndrome

52

Compartment syndrome (Fig. 52.1) is a very common complication following successful revascularization of arterial occlusion, which is why the indication for fasciotomy should be made generously from the outset. In contrast to chronic compartment syndrome, acute compartment syndrome is a clinical diagnosis. Instrumental measurement of compartment pressure can be performed as an adjunct, but the clinical findings are paramount.

Case Example
A 53-year-old man with a known intracardiac thrombus following myocardial infarction and ventricular aneurysm suffers an arterial embolism in the right leg. In the acute ischemia stage Rutherford IIb, an uncomplicated transfemoral embolectomy of the right superficial femoral artery and popliteal artery is performed, after which perfusion of the foot rapidly recovers. Due to the patient's age (cosmetic considerations in a relatively young man!) and his currently good condition, you consider whether a fasciotomy is necessary. What is your decision?

Definition
- Increase in pressure within the muscle compartments, usually in the extremities, almost exclusively in the lower leg, rarely in the upper extremity
- Overview of pressure values:
  - **<10 mmHg:** Normal value in adults
  - **10–20 mmHg:** slightly elevated pressure
  - **20–30 mmHg:** impending compartment syndrome
  - **>30–45 mmHg:** manifest compartment syndrome

Typical Patient
- Acute arterial occlusion under thrombolytic therapy or after successful surgical intervention

S. Regus, *Vascular Surgical Emergencies*,
https://doi.org/10.1007/978-3-662-72646-4_52

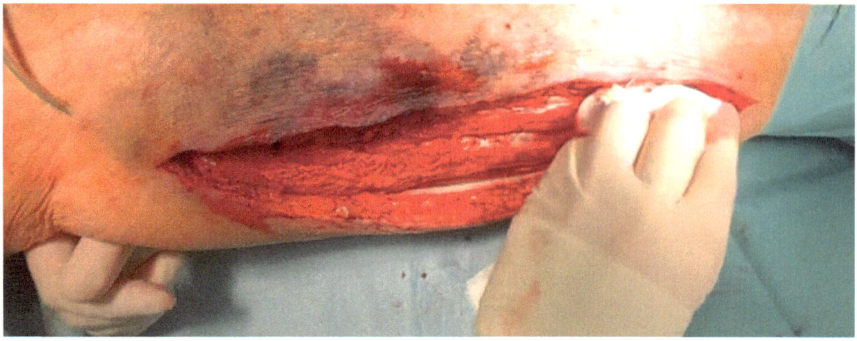

Fig. 52.1 Intraoperative finding of a fasciotomy for compartment syndrome of the lower leg

- Women without relevant pre-existing conditions after several hours of gynecological surgery in lithotomy position
- Polytraumatized patients with massive bleeding into the compartments (traumatic compartment syndrome)
- Status post successful resuscitation, often in the context of cardiogenic shock and myocardial infarction in patients with a corresponding cardiovascular risk profile and pre-existing pelvic/leg stenoses, which decompensate due to circulatory instability and, after normalization of circulation, cause a reperfusion syndrome

Typical On-Call Situation
- Patient from your own department under thrombolysis or after vascular surgery with increasing pain and a feeling of tension in the extremity. Here, however, it is important to distinguish bleeding from compartment syndrome.
- Pain in the lower legs and sensory deficits in the feet after several hours of gynecological surgery in lithotomy position
- Patient in the intensive care unit after resuscitation for myocardial infarction, now with pain and marked tension in one lower leg (rarely both)

Diagnostics
- Clinical examination
  - crucial
  - marked tenderness over the affected musculature, usually the anterior compartment
  - sensory loss between the first and second toe dorsally (compression of the deep peroneal/fibular nerve)
- If necessary, compartment pressure measurement
  - now available in many intensive care units
- Laboratory
  - CK, myoglobin, inflammatory markers

- Ultrasound
  - to differentiate compartment syndrome from hematoma

Therapy

- Conservative
  - Indications:
    with mild pressure increase <20 mmHg
    exclusion of arterial perfusion disorders
  - Approach:
    removal of constrictive dressings
    elevate the extremity (but not above heart level)
    correction of fluid and protein deficits
    close monitoring!
- Surgical
  - Indications:
    impending compartment syndrome and increasing pain
    manifest compartment syndrome
  - Approach:
    generous and prompt decision for fasciotomy
    opening of all 4 compartments of the lower leg from medial and lateral
    application of artificial skin (Epigard®) or a VAC dressing
    secondary closure only after significant reduction in swelling and tension-free skin adaptation

Call the on-call consultant at night?

- A manifest compartment syndrome must be urgently decompressed, so immediate contact is necessary—do not wait until the next morning.

Tips and Tricks

- Perform prophylactic fasciotomy directly during surgical management of an acute arterial occlusion, especially from Rutherford IIa onwards
- Do not forget neurolysis of the tibial nerve:
  - For this, the soleus arch, i.e., the fascia at the edge of the soleus muscle, must be incised
  - This relieves the tibial nerve
  - A partially closed fasciotomy is usually insufficient
- If necessary, use a primary adapting skin suture, which can later be removed on the regular or intensive care unit without new anesthesia if required
- Often, initial tamponade and coverage with artificial skin (Epigard®), followed by a VAC dressing the next day
- Compartment syndrome is a clinical diagnosis. Pain, tension, and beginning sensory disturbances are indications for surgical fasciotomy, even if compartment pressure measurements yield unremarkable values

Case Example Continued

You decide to perform a fasciotomy and, through a medial incision on the lower leg, open the superficial and deep flexor compartments, and through an incision lateral to the tibial crest, the peroneal and anterior compartments. The indication for fasciotomy should be made generously—better one time too often than too seldom. In cases of mild swelling, the skin can also be primarily sutured and, if swelling increases, the sutures can later be removed in the intensive care unit—without a new operation and without anesthesia.

GPSR Compliance

The European Union's (EU) General Product Safety Regulation (GPSR) is a set of rules that requires consumer products to be safe and our obligations to ensure this.

If you have any concerns about our products, you can contact us on ProductSafety@springernature.com

In case Publisher is established outside the EU, the EU authorized representative is:

Springer Nature Customer Service Center GmbH
Europaplatz 3
69115 Heidelberg, Germany

Batch number: 10726032

Printed by Printforce, the Netherlands